The Endometriosis
Natural Treatment Program

The Endometriosis Natural Treatment Program

A Complete Self-Help Plan
for Improving Health & Well-Being

Valerie Ann Worwood & Julia Stonehouse

New World Library
Novato, California

New World Library
14 Pamaron Way
Novato, California 94949

Abdominal cavity illustration on page 4 by Claire Thorne
Text design and typography by Tona Pearce Myers

Library of Congress Cataloging-in-Publication Data
Worwood, Valerie Ann.
The endometriosis natural treatment program : a complete self-help plan for improving health and well-being / Valerie Worwood and Julia Stonehouse.
    p.   cm.
Includes bibliographical references and index.
ISBN 978-1-57731-569-8 (pbk. : alk. paper)
1. Endometriosis — Popular works. 2. Endometriosis — Alternative treatment — Popular works. I. Stonehouse, Julia. II. Title.
RG483.E53W77 2007
618.1 — dc22   2006035824

First printing, June 2007
ISBN-10: 1-57731-569-3
ISBN-13: 978-1-57731-569-8

Printed in the United States on acid-free, partially recycled paper

g New World Library is a proud member of the Green Press Initiative.

10 9 8 7 6 5 4 3 2 1

The material in this book is not meant to take the place of a diagnosis and treatment by a qualified medical practitioner. Before making any decisions or taking any actions — or choosing, as a result of the material in this book, to undertake no action — consult with your physician or gynecologist. At the time of this writing, all information contained in this book is believed to be correct. Since the actual use of information contained in this book by a third party is beyond the authors' and publisher's control, no expressed or implied guarantee concerning its effects can be given nor liability taken, at any time, now or in the future, arising either directly or indirectly from reliance on the information, advice, or suggestions contained within this book, or in respect of any error or omission. Any application of the information set forth on the following pages is at the reader's sole discretion and risk, and the authors and publisher assume no responsibility for any actions taken either now or in the future.

This book is dedicated to Barbara Jean "Bobbie" Pilkington, whose
compassion and generosity of spirit touched so many

Sincere thanks to the Onaway Trust for their vision,
their understanding, and their support
of this natural treatment program

CONTENTS

PART TWO: THE NATURAL TREATMENT PROGRAM

A Blueprint for Success

Millions of women suffer from endometriosis, and their symptoms range from occasional discomfort to severe pain, along with other indicators that can persist for long periods and seriously impair their overall well-being and their family, professional, and social lives. If you are one of these women, you, like many others, may have found that conventional medical treatments offer limited relief at best. *The Endometriosis Natural Treatment Program* will help you take control of your endometriosis. This book focuses less on the problems of the condition than on the solutions, on making a series of slow, steady improvements that you yourself control.

The treatment program presented here was designed by one of the authors, Valerie Ann Worwood, a complementary-health practitioner and clinical aromatherapist who has shown that endometriosis can be treated in the context of a professional, holistic, complementary-medicine setting. For more than twenty years, she has used the plan to treat women of various ages and diverse cultures. All have experienced positive results, to differing degrees. Some followed the program to obtain relief while waiting for surgery, only to be told when the surgery took place that their endometriosis could no longer be found. Women with irregular menstrual cycles have found that the treatment plan has brought them into a regular cycle. It is not unusual for a woman following this program to become pregnant after having been told she was unlikely to conceive. These benefits stem from using this completely natural, noninvasive, simple set of lifestyle changes and procedures that can be carried out at home.

A brief version of this program appeared in *The Fragrant Pharmacy* (published in 1990 in the United States as *The Complete Book of Essential Oils and Aromatherapy*), a book that has subsequently been translated into several languages. We cannot know how many women with endometriosis have used the information in these books and benefited from it, but correspondence from all over the world has shown that many women have succeeded in using the suggestions to treat their own endometriosis.

In 1991, Valerie Ann Worwood adapted her treatment methods for a research trial with practitioners registered with the International Federation of Aromatherapists and women from the U.K. National Endometriosis Society. The trial set out to test the effectiveness of the method on women with endometriosis in reducing pain and other symptoms, as well as in improving general well-being. The participants in the study were carefully selected to exclude all other medical conditions and were precluded from using any other form of professional or self-help treatment during the twenty-four weeks of the trial: they could take no medications, nutritional supplements, or herbs, and could not use essential oils or undergo acupuncture or other complementary treatments that might confuse the trial results. Even though the trial used only one of the components of the self-help program given in this book, the results were impressive.

The program outlined on the following pages can be safely used with other medical treatments and is much more comprehensive than the version used in the research trial and the information provided in previous publications. This book presents and explains the many tools available to women who want to use natural methods to reduce the debilitating symptoms of endometriosis. It offers precise essential-oil formulations, self-massage techniques, and bath routines that, when carried out at home, appear to be effective in the treatment and management of endometriosis. The book offers recommendations for diet and lifestyle that reduce exposure to food compounds and environmental toxins that have been shown to exacerbate symptoms, and it emphasizes choices that boost the body's own defenses and healing processes. The program shows how self-massage, bodywork techniques, and exercise can help stimulate the body into self-healing. Finally, it outlines techniques for using essential oils, herbs, and homeopathic preparations that can be extremely effective in stimulating the body's own healing mechanisms.

Keeping detailed records of your symptoms, diet, activities, and treatment will help you monitor the effectiveness of your self-care program and supply valuable information to your physician and other health-care providers. Forms to help you with this record keeping are included in chapter 11.

The aim of the program is to trigger your body into behaving in a new way. In particular, the essential oils used in this program appear to help balance hormones and stimulate blood and lymphatic flow, thereby oxygenating the body, cleansing the tissues, and reducing inflammation and pain.

WHO IS THIS PROGRAM FOR?

This program is suitable for all women with endometriosis, no matter where they are on the usual treatment path. The program offers options whatever your circumstances, symptoms, and treatment history. For example, the program will be helpful for you if you

- have been recently diagnosed as having endometriosis;
- are taking medication for endometriosis;
- are considering taking medication for endometriosis;
- are considering surgery for endometriosis;
- have undergone surgery for endometriosis;
- have followed a course of medication and/or undergone surgery for endometriosis, without success;
- have discontinued your medication because of side effects;

- are currently using natural medication or treatment for endometriosis; or
- have endometriosis and have not yet followed any treatments, and would prefer to use natural methods as a first option.

Everything used in the program is derived from nature, and you can follow it alongside any other treatment you may be using. Every woman with endometriosis has a unique symptom profile, and not all the suggestions will be relevant to you. Many new treatment choices are presented here. You can select the ones best suited to you and form a complete plan for improving your health and well-being.

The next chapter offers an overview of researchers' current understanding of endometriosis, its symptoms, and its causes; this information is the basis of the natural treatment program.

PART ONE

Understanding Endometriosis

CHAPTER ONE

About Endometriosis

The name *endometriosis* comes from the word *endometrium*, the lining of the uterus. In endometriosis, tissue resembling uterine endometrial tissue is found outside the uterus — within the abdomen and elsewhere. Like tissue inside the uterus, endometrial tissue outside the uterus is thought to react to the hormonal signals of the monthly menstrual cycle, which act to build up tissue, break it down again, and eliminate it from the body by menstrual bleeding. However, unlike uterine tissue, which passes out of the body through the cervix and vagina, endometrial tissue in the abdominal cavity and elsewhere has no way to exit the body. Instead, it attaches to the lining of the abdomen or to other internal organs, often causing scar tissue or adhesions (abnormal tissue structures that bind organs or surfaces together).

Because endometrial cells can migrate within the body, endometriosis can develop anywhere within the pelvic or abdominal cavity. It is commonly found on the lining of the abdominal cavity (the peritoneum), on the ovaries, and on the outer surface of the uterus — especially the fundus (top), the right and left uterosacral ligaments, the right and left broad ligaments, the fallopian tubes, and the cul-de-sac (adjacent to the coccyx, or tailbone) — as well as on the bladder, the sigmoid flexure of the colon, the intestinal tract, the cervix, the vagina, the perineal area between the vagina and rectum, and even the vulva. Implanted endometrial tissue has also been found in the rectum and along surgical scars. Rarely, endometrial tissue is found outside the abdominal cavity — on the lung, eye, thigh, arm, and other sites.

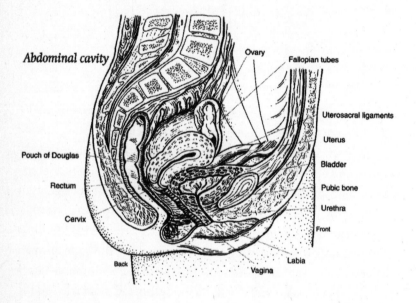

The implants can vary considerably in appearance, ranging from clear or grainy to white, reddish, brown, or blue-black. They can form into large cysts (endometriomas) attached to an ovary, some of which are termed "chocolate cysts" because of their dark blood color.

Endometrial cells can form a variety of implants, creating a condition medically categorized in four stages of severity:

1. Minimal disease: Top surface, or "superficial," implants, few in number, are present.
2. Mild disease: Deeper implants, greater in number, are present.
3. Moderate disease: Many implants are present. The ovaries are affected to some degree. Scar tissue, seen as filmy adhesions, is also present.

4. Severe disease: Many deep implants are present. Large endometriomas exist on one or both ovaries, along with scar-tissue adhesions.

Each woman's experience of endometriosis is unique. Some women may have extensive endometrial tissue but feel little or no pain, while other women may have only a few implants but feel tremendous pain. In other words, the degree of pain a woman experiences does not necessarily reflect the severity of her disease. This is one of the factors complicating endometriosis diagnosis and treatment.

DO YOU HAVE ENDOMETRIOSIS?

Researchers have estimated that it can take four to nine years for a woman with endometriosis to get a firm diagnosis. That's too long. Part of the difficulty, from a doctor's point of view, is that endometriosis has a huge number of possible symptoms, which vary in severity in every case.

Some women with endometriosis have no symptoms at all, and the condition is discovered only during a surgical procedure, such as sterilization, or during an examination into the cause of infertility.

Some women have pain only at certain times. For example, one of the most common sites of endometrial implants is on the uterosacral ligaments that hold the uterus in place. When the uterus is stimulated during intercourse, the woman might experience tremendous pain, although she may not experience it at other times.

Some women experience pain throughout the whole menstrual cycle, possibly because the endometrial implants or adhesions are located in sensitive areas.

SYMPTOMS OF ENDOMETRIOSIS

Some women have no symptoms, others have one or two, and some have many. The following is a list of possible symptoms, with the most common indicated by an asterisk.

- Abdominal and pelvic pain before, during, or after menstruation*

  - chronic pelvic pain
  - intermittent pelvic pain, either locally sharp or generalized
  - lower pelvic pain, from buttocks to groin
  - severe abdominal cramps
  - continual dull abdominal and/or backache

- Menstrual irregularities*

  - variable amount of bleeding, either heavy or scanty
  - premenstrual spotting
  - bleeding almost continuously over the month, or on a cycle lasting forty to sixty days
  - unpredictable occurrence and length of menstrual bleeding
  - blood clots

- Other pain, aches, and soreness

  - backache (especially before and during periods)*
  - pain in the coccyx*
  - pain in one or more joints
  - pain in the front of the thigh
  - headache
  - pain in the chest area
  - pain in the shoulder
  - pain around the rib cage (left, right, or both)
  - pain under the rib cage
  - pain in the rectum
  - pain upon tampon insertion

- Sexual and reproductive symptoms

  - pain during or after sexual intercourse (dyspareunia)*
  - infertility*
  - miscarriage
  - ectopic pregnancy

- Hormonal symptoms

  - hot flashes
  - tender breasts
  - PMS (premenstrual syndrome)

- Digestive symptoms

  - painful defecation*
  - bloating (often progressive over the course of the day)*
  - constipation (often because it hurts to pass stools)
  - rectal bleeding or blood in stools
  - diarrhea
  - sharp gas pains
  - fluid retention
  - nausea or vomiting
  - sugar craving
  - loss of appetite

- Urinary symptoms

  - irregular urination, either frequent or urgent, or retention of urine
  - lower abdominal pain on urination
  - blood in urine
  - kidney tenderness

- Cardiovascular symptoms

  - breathlessness
  - palpitations
  - giddiness
  - high blood pressure

- Mind, mood, and emotional states

  - depression
  - apathy, fatigue
  - poor concentration or memory
  - irritability

COMMON SYMPTOMS: A CLOSER LOOK

Abdominal Pain

Intense pain prior to and during menstruation is the most common symptom of endometriosis. The amount of pain felt largely depends on the location of the endometrial implants, the amount of scar tissue, and whether there are ovarian cysts or adhesions within the abdominal cavity, or internal bleeding.

In addition, endometrial cells and rupturing endometrial cysts release inflammatory chemicals, such as prostaglandins and histamine, that irritate pain receptors. Pain receptors affected by these chemicals become more sensitive with each successive exposure. Prostaglandin-induced uterine contractions in some women with endometriosis have been shown to equal or exceed in severity those of labor contractions in childbirth. Women who experience pain when not menstruating have described it as knifelike, sharp, or burning, particularly during ovulation.

Endometrial cells can also invade the tissues of other organs, causing their dysfunction and often additional pain. Moreover, the characteristic adhesions caused by endometrial implants can impede the flow of blood and oxygen to the affected organs, as well as trapping toxins. Unfortunately, even when the visible endometrial cells are surgically removed, the pain may persist.

Infertility and Miscarriage

Endometriosis is one of the main causes of female infertility. Several studies have shown that between 30 and 60 percent of women with endometriosis cannot conceive. The difficulties arise, first, from the physical damage any endometrial implants and scar tissue have caused to the reproductive organs, particularly the ovaries, fallopian tubes, and uterus. Hormonal imbalance disrupts the menstrual cycle, making ovulation uncertain or difficult to identify. And women who experience pain during intercourse tend to have sex less frequently, thus reducing their chances of conception. In addition, some of the medications used to treat the condition may impair fertility or conception.

Fertility is a mystery in the best of times, and even partners who seem to be in perfect reproductive health can have difficulty conceiving. There are many causes of infertility, including physical problems, hormonal imbalances, emotional issues, stress, nutritional deficiencies, side effects of medications, and chemical incompatibility between partners. It's no wonder that the precise effects of endometriosis on fertility have yet to be determined.

Pain during Intercourse (Dyspareunia)

When endometrial tissue is located in parts of the body that are stimulated during intercourse, it can cause intense pain. This is particularly the case when the uterosacral ligaments are affected.

HOW ENDO CAN AFFECT YOUR LIFE

Most people don't realize how severely endometriosis can affect a woman. Because the condition has a way of seeping into all aspects of life, it often leads to feelings of depression, low self-esteem, anxiety, and stress. When the endometriosis is undiagnosed, the sufferer may be accused of malingering or shunning her responsibilities. Even when the condition is diagnosed, a woman's family and friends may disbelieve the degree of pain she is experiencing. Women with daughters may feel further anxiety and guilt at the possibility of passing the condition on to them. The potential for experiencing debilitating pain at any time makes planning holidays and social events difficult. Sexual relationships are put under tremendous strain. All this can leave the sufferer feeling misunderstood and alone. In addition to the medical symptoms described above, other physical and psychosocial problems often affect women with endometriosis:

Premenstrual-type symptoms. Women with endometriosis may experience feelings of anger, hostility, irritability, and tiredness, as well as sugar cravings.

Difficulties at work. Women who are incapacitated by endometriosis for several days a month frequently suffer a loss of productivity and attendant loss of self-esteem, to say nothing of reduced chances of advancement. In some cases their absences may threaten their jobs. In addition, colleagues who do not understand the severity of the condition may suspect an endo sufferer of malingering and feel resentment toward her if they have to cover her work, straining work relationships and further contributing to the endo sufferer's feelings of isolation and depression.

Difficulties in personal relationships. The pain caused by endometriosis can impair sexual relationships. Intercourse is expected to lead to pleasure, not intense pain, and this conflict between expectation and actuality is often deeply disturbing to the male partner as well as to the woman. If a woman experiences pain with intercourse and has not been diagnosed with endometriosis, her partner might accuse her of being frigid or neurotic. This can lead to emotional and mental trauma, and even to the destruction of the relationship. Pain caused by endometriosis may also impair participation in other activities with one's partner, children, and friends, who may not be sympathetic if they do not fully understand the reason.

Loss of self-worth. A woman who cannot control her symptoms may feel a loss of control in other aspects of her life and a lack of self-confidence. She may also feel abnormal, isolated, and unfeminine. Moreover, if the woman lives in a culture where she is defined by her ability to produce children (and where a man's masculinity is defined by the number of children his wife produces), female infertility can also lead to a social stigma, resulting in divorce, social exclusion, and even suicide.

Difficulties with social life, plans, and travel. A woman whose symptoms are severe may have to plan holidays, family events, and other activities around her menstrual cycle.

Difficulties with spirituality and religious observance. Many religions and cultural traditions have taboos associated with menstruation. Some women whose menstrual bleeding is prolonged by endometriosis may find themselves frequently excluded from their places of worship, religious services, and other ceremonies and suffer further social exclusion as a result.

CHAPTER TWO

Securing an Accurate Diagnosis

Diagnosing endometriosis has proved difficult for the medical profession. Here we examine the main reasons and make some recommendations that may help you to obtain a timely and accurate diagnosis.

For many other conditions, definitive medical tests are available. For endometriosis, no such test exists, although there are certain biochemical "markers" that are more likely to be found in women with endometriosis. Inflammation, for example, can be assessed by looking for C-reactive protein (CRP) in the blood. But the only sure way to know if there are endometrial implants and scar tissue within the abdominal cavity is to perform a surgical procedure known as laparoscopy, in which a tiny camera is inserted into the abdomen through a small incision to allow visual inspection of the potentially affected areas.

From the pattern of symptoms, physicians can sometimes speculate where endometrial implants may be located. For example, vomiting and abdominal swelling can indicate implants on the small intestine. Pain when passing stools may indicate implants on the bowel. However, such speculation can be confirmed only by laparoscopy.

Some authorities suggest that the woman allow her physician to examine her at the height of her menstrual flow, when the endometrial implants in the abdominal cavity (as well as the endometrial cells within the uterus) are more swollen and therefore easier to detect. Although this process is not commonplace and may sound unpleasant, it is something you may wish to discuss with your physician.

BARRIERS TO DIAGNOSIS

The most common reasons women have difficulty securing an accurate diagnosis are as follows.

Some women do not provide their gynecologists with enough information about the full range of their specific symptoms. Anyone concerned with your condition, including you, has a better chance of understanding it, monitoring it, and treating it if he or she has a full and accurate picture of your physical and mental health, past and current treatments, diet, activities, and lifestyle. You can help in this by filling in the forms in chapter 11 and by keeping a daily diary of all your symptoms, including emotional states such as depression or anxiety.

It is particularly important to record abdominal pain. Measure each incident of pain in terms of the following:

- Duration
- Exact location in your body
- Severity, on a scale of one to ten, with ten being the worst
- Type: for example, sharp, dull, heavy

Also record all menstrual bleeding, noting:

- Duration (on the last day, record the number of days)
- Amount of flow
- The presence of clots

Record all other physical complaints, such as constipation, diarrhea, bloating, headaches, and nausea. If there is back pain or leg pain, identify the exact location. Also note any unusual appetite patterns or food cravings and any other symptoms (see above). It may be helpful to record any sexual activity as well.

All existing diagnostic procedures have significant disadvantages. Although laparoscopy is considered minor surgery, it is nevertheless an invasive procedure requiring scheduling, anesthesia, and recovery time. Ultrasound screening is noninvasive but less reliable.

Laparoscopy is relatively safe, but there have been a few cases where women suffered internal injury during the procedure, which led to the formation of scar tissue. It is usually carried out under a general anesthetic, although a few women opt for local anesthesia. Carbon dioxide is pumped into the abdominal cavity to separate the internal organs for clearer viewing. After the procedure, if some of this gas is left in the abdomen, it can cause pressure, usually perceived as shoulder pain, until it eventually disperses.

Ultrasound can be done in two ways. In transvaginal ultrasonography, or TVS, a small transducer is placed inside the vagina; in a transabdominal scan, it is placed on the lower abdomen. Another technique, color Doppler imaging (CDI), shows peripheral blood flow to the area. This is very helpful when trying to distinguish adenomyosis from fibroids (see pages 18–19). Ultrasound analysis should be done both before and after menstruation to detect changes in the activity of the ovaries or ovarian follicles. Changes in suspect tissue between the first and second scans allow physicians to distinguish between the presence of endometrial tissue and other disorders.

Nevertheless, endometriosis is difficult to diagnose with ultrasound alone, especially if there are no identifiable cysts or nodules of endometrial tissue. In women with stage 1 or 2 endometriosis, there may be only a few speckles of endometrial tissue, which do not show up with ultrasound. Similarly, small sheetlike areas will not be obvious.

Various other diagnostic tools are available to physicians. In culdocentesis, fluid is removed from the pelvic cavity, using a needle inserted through the vaginal wall, and tested for the presence of chemicals that indicate endometriosis. In cystoscopy, a thin fiberoptic tube is used to look inside the urethra, ureters, and bladder, and this procedure might be required in addition to laparoscopy if these areas are locations of problems that need exact interpretation. A hysteroscopy is a procedure that views inside the uterus and is useful for detecting adenomyosis, while hysterosalpingography detects problems with the fallopian tubes as well as the uterus.

Scan technology is improving all the time. Computed axial tomography (CAT or CT scanning) and magnetic resonance imaging (MRI) have recently been joined by electron-beam tomography (EBT), which can be very helpful in giving an overall picture of the abdominal area. The availability of these procedures depends on your locality and what you, your insurance company, or your national or local health authority are prepared to pay for.

The symptoms of endometriosis can be mistaken for those of another condition. The pain and other symptoms women experience with endometriosis are highly diverse, affecting many organs. When making a diagnosis, your physician will want to consider many other conditions and rule them out.

Other possible causes of endometriosis-type symptoms include the following:

- Specific conditions affecting the uterus, vagina, cervix, paracervix, fallopian tubes, ovaries, rectum, and urinary tract structures. These conditions may include fibroids, uterine prolapse, vestibulitis (pain in minor lips of vulva), ectopic pregnancy, ovarian cysts, ovarian cancer, bowel obstructions, inflammatory bowel disease, irritable bowel syndrome, and colon cancer.
- Specific conditions relating to the abdominal cavity and supporting structures, such as pelvic adhesions and hernia.
- Neurological problems in any of the above areas.
- Hormonal imbalances.
- Infections and inflammation, such as diverticulitis and pelvic inflammatory disease.
- Appendicitis.

- Adenomyosis, a condition involving endometrial implants in uterine tissue (see the sidebar "Adenomyosis: The Hidden Disease").
- Lesions.
- Sexually transmitted diseases, such as chlamydia and gonorrhea.

Because some of the above conditions are potentially life threatening, it's important to get an accurate diagnosis.

Both professionals and the public lack sufficient information about endometriosis. Endometriosis is still considered by some people to be just part of "a woman's lot," about which little can or needs to be done. Many older women remember a medical community that considered the symptoms of endometriosis as simply at the painful end of "normal" menstrual experience. Women used to be given no treatment other than painkillers.

A surprising degree of public ignorance of the condition also persists, despite the number of women affected. This may be partly because endometriosis has to do with the most private parts of the body, and sufferers do not like to talk about it to anyone other than close family and friends.

It is important to find specialists with detailed knowledge about the condition. Try to get a referral to a gynecologist specializing in endometriosis. Some diagnostic questions might be answered by an endocrinologist specializing in reproductive hormones.

Sometimes the degree of pain and discomfort a women suffers is not understood. In 1989, at the Second International Symposium on Endometriosis, Dr. W. Paul Dmowski delivered a paper saying that women with endometriosis are dismissed, devalued, and ignored (Halstead et al. 1989). Unfortunately, even today, many women suffer the same fate. If you find yourself in this position, exercise your right to see another health-care provider for a second opinion.

The amount of pain experienced does not directly indicate the amount of affected tissue. Depending on the location of the endometrial implants, some women with extensive endometriosis may feel no pain, while other women with only a few implants may feel a great deal of pain. Pain is therefore not a precise indicator of the extent of the condition. In some women, endometriosis quietly develops over a period of years and, by the time the woman is alerted to the problem, extensive scar tissue has formed. Conversely, a woman doubled up in pain for much of her life may find it is all due to a small implant in a troublesome position. The sheer variety of ways in which endometriosis presents itself makes diagnosis more difficult.

ADENOMYOSIS: THE HIDDEN DISEASE

Adenomyosis is a disease of the uterus that is sometimes confused with endometriosis. The name comes from *adeno*, meaning "gland," and *myosis*, meaning "muscle." In adenomyosis, endometrial tissue grows inside the muscular walls of the uterus, most commonly the back wall. This makes it impossible to see during a laparoscopy.

The symptoms of adenomyosis include abdominal pain and heavy or irregular bleeding during menstruation, but mild cases can be symptom free. Whereas endometriosis usually affects women between twenty and forty years of age, adenomyosis is more often diagnosed in older women. (This may simply be because it may take many years to diagnose. Often, it is diagnosed only retrospectively, after the uterus has been removed during a hysterectomy.) The uterus may appear lumpy during a laparoscopy and feel thick to the touch, and there may be a measurably increased flow of blood to the uterus, but the actual implants are not visible. For this reason, a woman with adenomyosis may be mistakenly diagnosed as having fibroids. Even in an ultrasound image, if the adenomyoses have clumped together into groups (known as adenomyomas), they can resemble fibroids. Color Doppler images (CDI) measuring blood flow are more helpful than ultrasound in detecting adenomyosis. A biopsy of uterine muscle can provide a definitive diagnosis.

Some women with endometriosis may also have adenomyosis. This explains why some women with few endometrial implants, as revealed by laparoscopy, still have considerable uterine pain and menstrual disruption.

Adenomyosis cannot be surgically corrected, but the size of the implants can sometimes be reduced through the use of laser fibers inserted into the muscle wall, guided by ultrasound imaging. Drug treatment includes anti-inflammatories and hormones (including birth control pills). An alternative option may be the Mirena IUD, an intrauterine device that slowly releases progesterone. This hormone thins the endometrium and reduces the volume of blood flow during menstruation. This IUD can be left in place for an extended period.

CHAPTER THREE

Causes of Endometriosis

All disease is perplexing. Why do some people get the flu when their family members and colleagues do not? Why, when two people eat the same contaminated food, might one person get food poisoning and the other not? In the case of endometriosis, the question might not be "Why does a particular woman develop endometriosis?" so much as "Why don't all women develop it?" There are at least ten reasons why a woman might develop endometriosis, and each woman's development and experience of the disease is probably the result of a unique and complex set of interacting factors. Some theories about the causes of the condition remain highly speculative.

The medical drug treatments for endometriosis reflect the general lack of understanding of its causes. For example, although physicians might agree that endometriosis sufferers have a hormonal imbalance, they may disagree about the nature of the imbalance: some prescribe synthetic testosterone (such as Danazol), while others prescribe a synthetic progesterone, medroxyprogesterone (such as Depo-Provera), and still others prescribe contraceptive pills that have differing ratios of estrogen and progesterone. In fact, the same physician might prescribe all of these hormone treatments to different women, or to the same woman at different times. There is no single ideal treatment, and physicians may offer a series of treatments in the hope that one of them will prove effective for the patient in question.

Each case of endometriosis is likely to be symptomatic of its unique set of causes. This is why it is so important to keep accurate records of your symptoms, diet, and daily activities. This information may reveal possible causes of your particular symptoms, and these, in turn, will help identify ways in which your treatment plan can be fine-tuned.

Many of the possible causes of endometriosis listed below may interact. They are grouped here into three general categories.

PHYSIOLOGICAL THEORIES

Retrograde Menstruation

The retrograde menstruation theory, first proposed by the New York physician John A. Sampson in 1921, suggests that, during menstruation, cells from the lining of the uterus (endometrial tissue) may fail to leave the uterus in the normal way, through the cervix and vagina. Instead they may travel in "retrograde" fashion through the fallopian tubes and adhere to the peritoneal surface or to the outer surface of pelvic structures such as the ovaries and uterus (Sampson 1927).

The fallopian tubes attach to the upper uterus, one on each side. At the point where the fallopian tubes narrow sharply at the uterine end are sphincter muscles. These are usually very tightly contracted. Normally, they relax at the time of ovulation, in response to the secretion of progesterone by the corpus luteum, permitting the release of the ovum from the ovary. Although it would seem very difficult for endometrial tissue to pass through the sphincter and the fallopian tube into the abdominal cavity, it might be possible during ovulation, when the sphincter is relaxed. Alternatively, perhaps some women produce too much progesterone, and the sphincter is slack much of the time, allowing tissue to pass through it.

There is some evidence both for and against this theory. Although it's well known that the exterior surface of the fallopian tube is a common site for endometrial implants, some experts have noted that the interior of the fallopian tubes is remarkably clear of endometrial tissue, especially during early stages of the disease. Others report that clearing the fallopian tube of "debris" has helped some women conceive.

Endometrial implants are often found on the ovaries. In 75 percent of all diagnosed cases of endometriosis, there is evidence of implants on one or both ovaries. This fact supports the retrograde menstruation theory, because the ovaries are right next to the openings of the fallopian tubes. Another suggestion is that loose endometrial tissue implants readily on the ovaries because they contain high levels of hormones.

Arguments against the retrograde menstruation theory mention the fact that inside the fallopian tubes there are millions of minuscule cilia (hairlike structures) whose job is to push the contents of the fallopian tubes toward the uterus rather than in the opposite direction. This motion helps a fertilized ovum to reach the uterus and implant itself. In addition, the muscles of the fallopian tubes contract occasionally — again, to help a fertilized egg reach the uterus. So, although retrograde menstruation may seem a logical cause for endometrial tissue ending up in the abdominal cavity, there are several anatomical reasons why this theory is difficult to prove.

How common is retrograde menstruation? We know this route is open in at least some women. Studies using X-rays taken after dye has been inserted into the uterus show the dye flowing backward through the fallopian tubes and into the abdominal cavity. Some other women have a mechanical defect or surgical scarring of the cervix. This inhibits normal menstrual flow, and blood and uterine tissue are known in some cases to escape backward, through the fallopian tubes. In other cases, an excess of prostaglandins can cause the cervix to tighten, preventing menstrual flow and possibly leading to retrograde menstruation.

How many women without these cervical problems experience retrograde menstruation, and how many develop endometriosis as a consequence, is a matter of intense debate. In a review of the available information, researchers concluded: "It is not proven that retrograde menstruation is a universal phenomenon occurring similarly with and without endometriosis" (D'Hooghe et al. 2002). Many statistics have been presented to suggest that all women have endometrial implants in the abdominal cavity to some extent. Robert Schenken, professor of obstetrics and gynecology at the University of Texas Health Science Center at San Antonio, found that, of women undergoing surgery for all gynecologic indications, only 1 percent of women had endometriosis. However, among women being examined surgically for pelvic pain, infertility, or dysmenorrhea, the figure rose to between 12 and 50 percent.

Intrauterine Migration

In some women, usually in their forties, the endometrial cells lining the womb push into the uterine muscles. This condition is known as adenomyosis (see the sidebar "Adenomyosis: The Hidden Disease" on pages 18–19). The cells do not migrate all the way into the abdominal cavity but remain embedded in the uterus. For this reason, these women do not have implants in the abdominal cavity or painful scar tissue. They may still have deep abdominal pain and heavier periods, but they do not have the same broad range of symptoms experienced by women with endometriosis.

Immune-System Factors

If endometrial tissue enters a woman's abdominal cavity, we would expect the immune system to destroy it. One theory of the development of endometriosis suggests that all women lose some endometrial tissue through retrograde menstruation, but in some women the immune system fails to destroy it.

This theory is supported by a survey of members of the Endometriosis Association in the United States, reported in the publication *Human Reproduction* in 2002 (17:2715). The research found that, among women with endometriosis, autoimmune inflammatory diseases were more common than in women without the condition.

There are several ways in which the immune system may affect endometrial cells in the abdominal cavity. The quantity of lymphocytes (white blood cells) or their antibodies may be reduced, or the lymphocytes may be unable to recognize the endometrial cells as misplaced. Another theory is that the increased number of lymphocytes needed to destroy the endometrial cells secrete sufficient toxins and growth factors into the peritoneal fluid that they actually stimulate the growth of endometrial tissue. Another hypothesis is that the affected tissues are insufficiently oxygenated, allowing the inflammation to continue unabated.

Inflammation

Endometriosis is known to have an inflammatory component; the question is whether the inflammation is the cause of endometriosis or the consequence of it. In *The Inflammation Cure* (2003), Dr. William Joel Meggs outlines his belief that inflammation within the body may be at the root of many diverse conditions, from heart disease to obesity, and from Alzheimer's to osteoporosis.

Inflammation is part of the immune system's work of destroying invading microorganisms or toxic substances and repairing damaged tissue. It should occur in an acute situation, as a temporary step in our body's defenses to get us over a crisis, but, Meggs speculates, more and more often the inflammation is chronic, or ongoing.

Inflammation can be triggered by both the immune system and the nervous system. In asthma, for example, which involves inflammation of the breathing apparatus, an attack can be brought on both by environmental factors, such as vehicle emissions, and by emotional trauma.

The world we live in today is very different from the environment in which humans first evolved, and, according to the inflammation hypothesis, the human immune system has not yet caught up with the changes. It is struggling to deal with the chemical onslaught we are all exposed to: environmental pollutants in the air we breathe, in the food we eat, in the products we put on our bodies, in our homes and gardens, and in our workplaces. All these compounds put stress on the immune system and may cause inflammation.

In addition, whereas the nervous system was originally adapted to respond to sudden, intermittent stresses (as when a herd of buffalo approached at a gallop, for example), we are now exposed to stress just by hearing the daily news and managing our hectic lives.

For a woman with endometriosis, it's important to understand that stress, like environmental pollutants, can cause inflammation. Whether it's a cause or effect of endometriosis, inflammation is painful, and reducing it must be a priority. The first, most obvious step to take is to minimize exposure to environmental and emotional stressors.

Levels of inflammation can be tested by measuring the C-reactive protein (CRP) in the blood. You might consider having your CRP checked before and after carrying out any program of detoxification and/or stress reduction. Afterward you can ask yourself: Has the inflammation level gone down? And how are the symptoms, especially the pain?

LYMPHATIC OR VASCULAR TRANSPLANTATION THEORY (METASTASIS)

This theory suggests that endometrial cells from the uterus travel in either the lymph or the blood circulatory systems and are deposited in the abdominal cavity. This hypothesis arises from the observation that endometrial tissue is occasionally found outside the abdominal area — for example, in the lungs, liver, gallbladder, stomach, and spleen. Endometrial tissue has even been discovered in skin, armpits, and eyes. This theory offers an explanation of how it gets there.

However, as endometrial tissue is only rarely found in the lymph nodes, which is where it would normally accumulate and be dealt with if it traveled through the lymphatic system, it seems unlikely that it does so. Whether endometrial cells travel in the blood should be easy enough to discover, especially given the new diagnostic tool of live blood analysis, but research in this area has yet to be carried out.

Iatrogenic Origins

Iatrogenic means "physician-produced": that is, inadvertently caused or aggravated by some form of medical intervention. The theory of iatrogenic transplantation suggests that, during a surgical procedure, cells from the internal wall of the uterus might be transferred on surgical equipment to the abdominal cavity, where they adhere to the surface of the peritoneum or to an organ within the cavity. In a very few cases, endometriosis might have been caused in this way — for example, during a cesarean section or episiotomy.

In a few other cases, it seems possible that endometriosis was caused by prescription medications. These are not common incidents, but women should be aware of them and discuss them with their health-care providers.

Dr. Ellen Grant, in her book *Sexual Chemistry*, argues that, although most contraceptive pills thin the endometrial lining of the uterus, they also cause the blood vessels to distort and dilate, which may cause the endometrial tissue to move backward through the veins. If this is the case, although the pill may reduce the profuse monthly bleeding experienced by some women, when the pill is stopped, the misplaced tissue "thickens and bleeds more profusely," leading to the diagnosis of endometriosis (Grant 1994).

Another concern was raised by a letter to the *British Medical Journal*, in which Dr. John Svigos reported that the antiestrogen drug Clomid (clomiphene citrate), used to treat infertility, caused 57 percent of women to develop endometriosis, compared with 7 percent in the control group (Svigos 1990).

For women who already have endometriosis, a worrying piece of research carried out on baboons by Dr. Thomas D'Hooghe and associates showed that "immunosuppression may increase the incidence of endometriosis in baboons with spontaneous disease"

(D'Hooghe 1995). (*Spontaneous* in this context refers to baboons that have endometriosis naturally.) The drugs used in the trial were the corticosteroid IM methylprednisolone and the antirheumatic drug azathioprine.

Corticosteroids are commonly used to treat rheumatoid arthritis, systemic lupus, asthma, inflammatory skin conditions, psoriasis, eczema, dermatitis, inflammatory bowel disease, and certain connective tissue disorders, and, in conjunction with azathioprine, to prevent rejection after organ transplants. They are also sometimes included in skin preparations for skin ulcers, burns, wounds, and even diaper rash. They work by blocking the prostaglandins that trigger an inflammatory response, particularly following tissue damage. They also suppress allergic reactions and immune-system activity. This research raises the question, Do certain anti-inflammatory drugs stimulate the growth of endometriosis in women, as they do in baboons?

Coelomic Metaplasia

Embryological studies have shown that all organs in the pelvis (including the endometrium) originate as cells of the peritoneal-abdominal (coelomic) cavity lining. The term *metaplasia* refers to any type of tissue transforming into another type. The coelomic metaplasia theory of endometriosis proposes that some of the cells of the peritoneum (the abdominal wall) develop into endometrial cells instead of normal peritoneal cells, or instead of the usual cells that make up the organs within the abdomen. The cause may be irritation from retrograde menstruation, from chronic infection or inflammation, or from overexposure to hormones or chemicals.

This theory was first given support by a scientific paper published in 1971, reporting the case of a man who developed endometriosis in his bladder following treatment for prostate cancer using estrogenic drugs (Oliker and Harries 1971). Several similar cases have been reported since.

The endometriosis found in these men clearly did not come from uterine tissue. It had to come from somewhere, and the metaplasia theory currently offers the only explanation.

CONGENITAL OR EMBRYONIC REST THEORY

Another theory involving irregular cellular development suggests that, during the embryonic stage, some endometrial cells that should grow in the womb instead develop in the abdomen. They are then activated in puberty under the influence of the hormones estrogen and progesterone.

Hormonal Factors

Both the male and the female body develop with the appropriate balance of hormones. We have come a long way in our understanding of the number and complexity of human hormones. The idea that the male has testosterone and the woman has estrogen and progesterone is now seen as simplistic. Men and women have the same hormones, but we have them in different ratios and strengths. In women, hormones are present in varying quantities depending on such factors as age, the menstrual cycle, and reproductive status.

Endometriosis occurs during a woman's reproductive years, when ovarian hormones, including estrogen and progesterone, are most active in her body. Because endometriosis does not generally occur before puberty or after menopause, it's clear that hormones play a role in its development. One suggestive sign is that women with endometriosis generally start menstruating at an earlier age. Any woman who suspects she has endometriosis should be tested for all reproductive hormone levels, especially if her physician intends to prescribe hormone-manipulating drugs.

Estrogen has many functions within the female body, including making the uterine lining thicken so that it is prepared to accept a fertilized egg. It is also said to exacerbate the activity of endometrial implants. Most drug treatments for endometriosis aim, in one way or another, to reduce the production of estrogen. Unfortunately for a woman trying to conceive, these treatments involve trying to mimic one of the states during which estrogen levels are low: pregnancy or menopause. Estrogen-reducing drug treatments will cause difficulty in conceiving, and if conception does occur, the drugs may be harmful to the baby's development.

Progesterone counters some of the effects of estrogen and is sometimes called the "pregnancy hormone." Progesterone levels increase during ovulation and dramatically during pregnancy (from the normal twenty milligrams a day to as much as four hundred milligrams a day). One of its effects is to slow endometrial growth; another is to render the uterine muscle inactive (so that the developing fetus is not prematurely expelled by contractions). Medical treatments for endometriosis often try to mimic "the progesterone effect" to fool the body into thinking it's pregnant. The difficulty with all progesterone-based treatments (and progesterone-heavy diets) is that they can make it difficult for a woman to conceive.

Prostaglandins are the hormones thought to cause the pain of endometriosis. They are so called because, when first identified in 1935, they were thought to be produced only by the male prostate. We now know that there are at least twenty varieties, and many more may be discovered since they are found in almost every human cell. The particular prostaglandin involved in endometriosis is called F2-alpha, and one of its roles is to stimulate uterine contractions.

When it's produced in a reasonable quantity, F2-alpha is a helpful hormone because it causes menstrual fluid to be expelled from the uterus each month. However, when produced in excess, it not only causes terrible cramping, but it can also make the cervix contract so that the menstrual flow cannot escape. If this happens, the prostaglandin is absorbed by the tissues of the uterus, causing even more cramping and pain.

There are many other hormones involved in the female reproductive cycle, and they must all be kept in balance. Testosterone is

produced by the ovaries as well as by the adrenal glands. Possibly significant in the development of endometriosis are the hormones that
trigger the production of estrogen: follicle-stimulating hormone
(FSH), which in turn is stimulated by gonadotropin-releasing hormone (GnRH). These are regulated by the pituitary gland and hypothalamus, respectively, so the action of these crucial structures
deep inside the brain may play a part in the development of endometriosis.

Genetic Factors

It's long been known that genes play some role in endometriosis, as
it often runs in families. A study of 719 women in Utah with surgically
diagnosed endometriosis confirmed that there is a genetic element to
endometriosis. In 2001 an even larger survey was carried out by the
National University Hospital in Iceland, which looked at the records
of 750 Icelandic women who had surgery for endometriosis between
1981 and 1993, as well as examined a genealogical database for Iceland's entire population of about 290,000 people. This study found
that a woman is five times more likely than average to have endometriosis if her sister has it and 50 percent more likely to have it if
a female cousin has it.

Iceland's remarkable database offers an excellent possibility of
identifying the gene that predisposes certain women to develop endometriosis. In the meantime, women who have endometriosis in
the family may want to consider starting their families earlier in their
reproductive years, as the condition invariably gets worse over time,
and to embark on a preventive plan, one that includes many elements
of this natural treatment program.

ENVIRONMENTAL THEORIES
Xenoestrogen Overload

The human body absorbs hundreds of chemicals from the environment. Today these include xenoestrogens, synthetic chemicals that

mimic naturally occurring estrogen. They are not produced deliberately but are present as by-products of manufacturing processes. For example, xenoestrogens may leach out of plastic water bottles.

The effect of these xenoestrogens on the body is a subject of intense debate. The discussion largely focuses on observations of the increasing feminization of certain animals, including humans, in recent decades. The genitals of male alligators have become deformed; the testicles of more and more boys fail to descend. Sexual development, which is stimulated by hormones, is being disrupted across species.

An overload of xenoestrogens may stimulate the growth of endometrial tissue and cause endometriosis. It may also interact with other potential causes of endometriosis listed here, especially hormonal factors, coelomic metaplasia, congenital or embryonic rest theory, and environmental toxins.

Environmental Toxins

In the early 1970s, as part of an investigation into reproduction, a group of rhesus monkeys were exposed to the environmental pollutants 2,3,7,8-tetrachloro-dibenzo-p-dioxin and PCBs (polychlorinated biphenyls). Endometriosis developed in 79 percent of monkeys who were exposed, and in only 33 percent of monkeys who were not.

Many studies have shown that the average human body absorbs hundreds of synthetic chemicals from the environment. These chemicals come from all kinds of things: insecticides, herbicides, fungicides, food and drink, food packaging, gasoline, household cleaning products, dry-cleaning chemicals, cosmetics, personal care products, and the air we breathe. They rise in unseen clouds from new carpeting and building materials. When we fill a car's gas tank, a benzene cloud forms from the nozzle like a naughty genie from a bottle.

We spray synthetic fragrances on our necks and rub a cocktail of chemicals on our bodies. If you look at the ingredients of your skin care products, you will likely find one or more of the following: methyl paraben, propyl paraben, benzyl paraben, ethyl paraben, and isobutyl paraben. Parabens have been linked to the development of breast cancer and have been shown to have an estrogenic effect in animal uterine tissue. Personal care products contain many other synthetic ingredients that may be absorbed into the body, perhaps only in tiny amounts. We don't know what effect these synthetic components may have on our bodies or on the development of endometriosis.

Although precisely measuring exposure to and effects of this daily chemical cocktail is impossible, research does show that this overload may increase our exposure to free radicals, which are believed to cause uncontrolled cellular growth. If endometriosis is a disease of misplaced or inappropriate cellular growth, synthetic chemicals may contribute to it.

OTHER THEORIES

There is still a great deal of speculation about the cause or causes of endometriosis. Theories abound. Examination of peritoneal fluid shows that women with endometriosis have higher concentrations of certain hormones and other natural chemicals. Among those under discussion are macrophage migration inhibitory factor, PP14, CA-125, CD2, CD4, CD8, interleukin (IL)2R, serum IL-6, and PF TNF-alpha, some of which have been implicated in other medical conditions. Another subject of inquiry is certain antigens and antibodies that are found in women with endometriosis but not in healthy women. These discoveries may lead to the development of diagnostic tools, but it will take longer to discover whether they lead to an effective treatment.

Although women with endometriosis might sometimes think that no medical research is being done into their condition, there has been a great deal of basic scientific investigation on the subject. The problem is that, when it's ascertained that a woman with endometriosis has a higher concentration of a particular chemical in her peritoneal fluid, the question remains whether that abnormality is a cause or an effect of the disease. Overproduction of a certain natural chemical may stimulate the growth of endometrial implants, or the endometrial implants themselves may secrete the chemical under study.

Despite much scrutiny of the problem, medical science still cannot come up with a definitive answer for the woman who asks, "Why me?" Consequently, women anxious to find *some* explanation for their condition may start blaming themselves. They may fear, for example, that having sex during menstruation, using tampons, eating the wrong foods, or working in an unhealthy environment is to blame. Here are a few of the possibilities that have been brought up, not necessarily as a cause of endometriosis, but as potential contributing factors:

Sex during Menstruation

It has been suggested that intercourse or orgasm during menstruation might force the endometrial tissue into the fallopian tubes. There is no scientific evidence for this view. If some women have a tendency to lose endometrial tissue through the fallopian tubes, this type of sexual activity may exacerbate it, but we do not know.

Tampon Use

There does not seem to be any reason to suppose that tampons increase the risk of endometriosis. In fact, some research has suggested they might be helpful, as they draw menstrual blood away from the uterus. However, most tampons (and pads, for that matter) are made with bleached material. The bleaching process produces dioxins, which are already implicated in the development of endometriosis (see above).

Douches

No link has ever been made between the use of douches and the development of endometriosis. Most women use just plain water. However, it would probably be wise not to douche with any synthetic products, given the fact that the vaginal mucous membrane is an extremely absorbent surface.

Baths

If chemical bath products are used regularly, and if the water enters the vagina during bathing (which is usual), then perhaps these chemicals are being absorbed through the delicate vaginal mucous membrane and affecting the reproductive organs. No products have yet been implicated in this potential route of absorption. However, it may be something to think about.

Sexually Transmitted Diseases

There has never been a suggestion that sexually transmitted diseases cause endometriosis. There just does not seem to be a link. Pelvic inflammatory disease might exacerbate scar tissue development, but it is very unlikely that it causes endometriosis.

Stress and Emotional Factors

One of the foremost researchers into the mind-body connection, Candace Pert, has said that "your mind is in every cell of your body" (1997). This was not a vague statement but an observation based on intense scientific study. Because receptors for certain brain chemicals are found not only in the brain itself but also in the immune system, the nervous system, and the endocrine system, there is no physical distinction between the mind and the body. Stress and emotions stimulate brain chemicals and, it seems, physically affect the immune system and endocrine systems — both of which are implicated in the development of endometriosis.

Stress may directly affect the body in other negative ways, some of which may exacerbate endometriosis. For example, cortisol, a steroid produced by the adrenal glands, is produced in response to stress, and it may affect the liver function and the types of cholesterol we produce. This, in turn, may affect the body's ability to clear toxins, such as those that may stimulate the growth of endometriosis.

Nutrition

Nutrition comes into the discussion of endometriosis for at least three reasons. First, good nutrition keeps the immune system working well. Second, we can choose to keep our intake of potentially harmful chemicals to a minimum by eating organic, unprocessed foods. Third, certain compounds in plants we eat have qualities very similar to those of human hormones; these are said to have phyto-hormonal effects (*phyto* means leaf, thus "of the plant").

For example, compounds known as lignans, which have an estrogenic effect, are found in high levels in flaxseed, broccoli, asparagus, carrots, and squash. Lower amounts are also present in nuts, berries, whole grains, and various other oil-bearing seeds. Because lignans bind to estrogen receptors, albeit weakly, they prevent the estrogen produced by the body from binding to those receptors. Ironically, then, a small estrogenic effect from these foods results in an overall reduction in estrogen uptake. In addition, lignans inhibit the action of aromatase, an enzyme that converts testosterone into estrogen.

If high levels of estrogen are associated with endometriosis, and lignans inhibit the effect of human estrogen and even synthetic xenoestrogens, lignans should be a useful component of the diet of a woman with endometriosis.

CELLS: THE BUILDING BLOCKS OF HEALTH

Endometriosis and adenomyosis are diseases of the cells. For reasons not yet understood, they develop in some women and not in others. In endometriosis the cells develop within the abdominal cavity, and in adenomyosis they develop inside the uterine muscle wall. The question is, why do these cells behave incorrectly? What sets them off? Do they replicate or die at the wrong time? Is it something to do with the chemistry of the cells, or their electrical energy, or their polarity? Are they deficient in some element they require in order to work correctly? Or is the source of the problem far away, in a gland, the pancreas, or the liver — which are, of course, made up of more cells?

Each of the fifty trillion or so individual cells in the human body is a miracle, an unbelievably complex and productive unit, assigned a specialist function. There are hundreds of different types of cells. Each contributes in its own way to the processes that sustain life: extracting energy and essential chemical inputs from food, distributing it to the right places, protecting against harmful microorganisms and substances, and removing waste. The job of the cells in your heart, for example, is to pump between eight thousand and forty thousand liters of blood a day — depending on whether you are lying on the sofa or running a marathon.

There is a constant flow of communication both among the different components within the cell and between cells. It takes place by means of countless trillions of chemical and electrical signals, switches, and reactions. Tiny disruptions of these processes may lead to malfunction and disease; conversely, tiny adjustments may improve cellular function and overall health.

Cells are constantly building themselves up, disintegrating, and being built up again into new cells. Every day, billions of cells go through programmed cell death, or apoptosis. Their "lifespan" ranges from less than an hour to more than a month. Some cells, however, don't die at the right time. They might die prematurely when attacked by a bacterium or toxin. They might just hang around and refuse to die, or they might go into a frenzy of reproduction, dividing and proliferating. Either way, disrupted cellular activities can cause cancer and other physical difficulties.

Each cell is encased by a plasma membrane, physically strong but flexible. The membrane has many different chemical "doors" that allow raw materials, fuel, and certain messenger molecules to enter, and manufactured proteins and waste material to pass out. Normally, foreign materials such as viruses and toxins are detected by their chemical structure and blocked from entering the cell. Some, of course, make it through and cause damage.

There are receptors on cell walls that pick up a chemical message and transduce it, or translate it, into a signal that is received within the cell, stimulating it to behave in a certain way. Some cells are instructed by hormones like estrogen, progesterone, testosterone, epinephrine (adrenaline), and insulin. They transmit messages from glands, such as the pituitary, hypothalamus, and adrenal glands. Of particular interest in endometriosis are the two receptors coded to respond to estrogen, known as ER-α and ER-β. These two receptors, which may have differing functions, respond not only to the estrogen generated within the body but also to phytoestrogens (from plants) and endocrine-disrupting chemicals (xenoestrogens). These responses may hold clues to the causes of and treatments for endometriosis.

Oxygen is vital to cellular processes. However, in the form of rogue oxygen molecules called free radicals it can also react chemically in harmful ways with all parts of the cell, including the proteins that form the inner structures of the cell and the DNA that contains the information essential to cell replication. Antioxidant compounds, such as those found in various plants, are beneficial because they protect against these damaging intracellular reactions.

The chemical processes within cells produce waste

products such as carbon dioxide and urea, which must be removed from the cell. The body also has to deal with the waste from worn-out cells. If the cells' organizational or cleansing systems are not working well, some waste molecules accumulate inside cells, unable to move. The cells can become clogged up and cease working efficiently.

If you think of a cell as a city, then you may recognize that, in order for that city to remain in good working order, it needs regular maintenance and repair. Sometimes it's useful to give your cells a little help. Supplements such as vitamins, minerals, and tissue salts give your cells materials they need to repair themselves. It's also important to minimize cell damage caused by inhaled or ingested toxins, such as those from cigarettes, alcohol, or chemical additives in food. Reducing emotional stress can help control negative changes within your own natural chemical environment. When trying to undertake a body maintenance and repair program, as you are now, it is essential to give the cells all the help you can and to allow them to function at their best.

CHAPTER FOUR

The Importance of a Holistic Health Approach to Endometriosis

We have seen that there are multiple reasons why endometriosis might develop but that researchers cannot pinpoint specific causes or triggers. Scientific research depends on slow, painstaking isolation and testing of cause and effect. Until the root causes of endometriosis are better understood, this treatment plan recommends taking all approaches simultaneously to try and defeat it, whatever the cause. We can do so by minimizing our exposure to manageable risk factors, by using natural methods to ease pain and other symptoms, and by using various natural therapies to heal and strengthen our bodies.

Most of the supposed causes of endometriosis may interact with each other to some extent. The two exceptions are iatrogenic transplantation and genetic factors. The following list traces the possible interactions.

- Retrograde menstruation

    - May stimulate coelomic metaplasia.
    - May be caused by overproduction of progesterone.

- Immune system factors

    - A weak immune system cannot clean up cells misplaced by retrograde menstruation.

❖ A weak immune system cannot effectively deal with dioxins and other environmental toxins.

- Inflammation

  ❖ May be caused by retrograde menstruation.
  ❖ May be uncontrolled because of weakened immune system.
  ❖ May be caused by the body's attempts to deal with xenoestrogen overload.
  ❖ May be caused by the body's attempts to deal with environmental toxins.

- Lymphatic or vascular transplantation

  ❖ More likely if the immune system is weakened.
  ❖ More likely if birth control pills (see iatrogenic origins) do cause dilation of veins and movement of endometrial tissue into the veins.

- Iatrogenic origins

  ❖ Anti-inflammatories used to treat chronic infection or inflammation may stimulate coelomic metaplasia.
  ❖ Birth control pills stimulate hormonal factors.

- Coelomic metaplasia

  ❖ May be caused by retrograde menstruation.
  ❖ May be caused by inflammation.
  ❖ May be caused by hormonal or anti-inflammatory treatments (see iatrogenic origins).
  ❖ May be caused by xenoestrogen overload.
  ❖ May be caused by environmental toxins.

- Congenital or embryonic rest theory

  ❖ Possibly stimulated by naturally occurring hormonal imbalance.
  ❖ Possibly stimulated by hormonal medications.

- Hormonal factors
  - Hormonal imbalance may be caused by hormonal medications.
  - Hormonal imbalance may be caused by xenoestrogen overload.
- Xenoestrogen overload
  - May be exacerbated by overload of naturally produced estrogen.
  - May stimulate coelomic metaplasia.
- Environmental toxins
  - May weaken the immune system.
  - May transform cells, stimulating coelomic metaplasia.
  - May disturb hormonal balance.

Given all the possible causes of endometriosis and the complicated ways in which they might interact, it seems fruitless to focus on any single cause or treatment. Moreover, most of the conventional therapies available are imperfect remedies. Although many women have found relief from their symptoms with drug treatments, there is a high incidence of recurrence: when a woman stops taking the drugs, the symptoms return. The drugs currently available have little effect on adhesions, and they may have unpleasant or debilitating side effects. Surgery carries the risk of damaging tissue and organs and causing additional scarring or adhesions. Also, surgery may fail to detect and remove all endometrial implants, so symptoms may persist. One area where implants cause a lot of pain, and where they are very difficult to see or work on surgically, is the area between the cervix and rectum, known as the "pouch of Douglas." Another difficulty is that endometrial implants can form thin sheets of tissue: these may be too indefinite to show up on ultrasound and yet too large to remove with laser therapy. Consequently, even the most advanced medical therapies prescribed by the most dedicated physicians may not bring complete or lasting relief from endometriosis.

Holistic treatment offers a different approach. It sees the body as a whole, integrated system, with each part and system having a direct effect on all others. If one part of the system is out of sync, other parts will be, too. Holistic practitioners seek to make connections between symptoms and use techniques and natural products that may have a healing effect on several systems at the same time.

The natural methods used in this program don't cause side effects. They interact well with each other, and most can be integrated with conventional medicine. Of course, it would be satisfying to understand exactly why the program is so effective, but at the end of the day, this doesn't matter to women with endometriosis as much as the fact that it works.

PART TWO

❧

The Natural Treatment Program

CHAPTER FIVE

Inner Preparation for the Endometriosis Natural Treatment Program

Many people don't take endometriosis seriously, perhaps because it's not life threatening and they can't imagine how painful it can be or how it can devastate a woman's life. Perhaps they believe the pain of endometriosis is no worse than that of a really bad period. How many times have you heard "It can't be that bad," or "It's normal — all women get pain," or "She's putting it on." Unless you're laid up for fifteen days of the month, people think you're all right — they can't see the pain or the anguish.

Endometriosis involves places so intimate we don't want everyone to know about it. Many women hide the fact that they have endometriosis, even from their partners, friends, work colleagues, and bosses. They suffer in silence, isolated. Medical attitudes vary a lot. In some countries, endometriosis is not identified as such and the symptoms are accepted as part of a woman's inevitable fate of suffering. Even in some modern, industrialized countries, it can still take years to get a diagnosis — six years is average in the United Kingdom, for example.

In an ideal world, women would be swiftly diagnosed by aware and up-to-date medical practitioners, who would perform a barrage of preliminary tests — for hormone levels, for example — and explain to their patients all the possible treatment options and their potential side effects. In reality, many women with endometriosis have to struggle for understanding, diagnosis, and a cure.

If your endometriosis has been diagnosed for a few years, you've likely been offered a series of drugs, one after the other. You may feel like a laboratory guinea pig: examined, evaluated, experimented on — and exhausted! How many times must a woman put up with having her feet in stirrups on the examination table, with being an object of speculation? How many times must her insides be prodded, scraped, laser-treated, and burned? Strangers know more about your ovaries than you do, because they view the laparoscopic images while you lie sedated and unable to move, let alone see anything. You have probably become an expert on painkillers that no longer work.

A woman with endometriosis can't be discreet about her sexual body and must lay it open like a book for the medical profession to read. She cannot be demure when her abdominal pain, urination patterns, bloating, bleeding, clots, and even fecal movements are a matter of general discussion. When sexual intercourse is painful, she cannot always be the willing, relaxed lover she would like to be. And finally, the ultimate cruelty, she may be unable to conceive, and never will conceive while taking some of the standard drugs for endometriosis, because they put the female body into a state of pseudo-pregnancy or pseudomenopause. For many sufferers, endometriosis is an affront to the female experience on all levels.

Endometriosis is not life threatening, but it is life interrupting. It's difficult to plan holidays when you know there will be long periods of time when you are too incapacitated to get on a plane. Even a nice evening out with friends might have to be cut short if the pain gets too bad. You never know when pain is going to strike. It's merciless, tiresome, and, for many women, ongoing.

You might be familiar with all of the above, or just some of it, but the fact that you are reading this indicates you're seeking an alternative to your current healing program. Perhaps you have only just been diagnosed and are looking at your options. Perhaps you want to try something entirely natural before going down the drug-therapy-and-surgery route, or maybe you have tried drug treatments already and they did not suit you. Perhaps you want to do something for yourself while, at the same time, following the drug treatment prescribed by your gynecologist.

One group of women whom the self-help program outlined here will certainly interest are those who want to get pregnant, but who have been told that most of the available drug therapies do make it far more difficult to conceive.

Each woman has a unique experience with endometriosis. Her set of symptoms is unique, and her personal circumstances differ from those of other women, such as her partner's attitude and her friends and family support system. Each individual woman will have to look at the following program and ask, "Is this for me?"

This self-help program involves an effective combination of disciplines. Some are therapeutic in the sense that they involve the use of essential oils or nutritional or herbal supplements. Some elements involve changes in your diet and in your personal care products, cosmetics, and household products in order to eliminate your exposure to potentially harmful ingredients. And the program also contains important elements that relate to your mental and emotional approach — so, before starting the self-help program outlined in the following chapter, think about the inner path to wellness.

THE INNER PATH TO WELLNESS

Gain Control

Taking control of your condition means an end to feeling helpless. It's easy to accept whatever physicians tell us, and as time goes on we may develop the feeling that we're on a roller coaster made up of other people's attempts to solve the problem. You will feel less helpless if your physician discusses your options fully. Even if you have a good relationship with your gynecologist, question everything — this is your right — and get second opinions. If you inquire, you will find information that will help you take control of your condition. Be sure to write down all your questions before consulting your physician: it's easy to forget them during the consultation itself.

The self-help program outlined on these pages gives you the information you need in order to take control of your own body. The hardest part of the program may be adopting the frame of mind that allows you to actually do so.

Don't Feel Guilty

It is not your fault that you are unwell. As we have seen, there are so many possible causes of endometriosis that the question is not "Why me?" but "Why not everyone?" Millions of women have endometriosis, and it's not their fault either.

An entire industry has grown up around the "you make yourself ill" school of thought. But things just happen, and different things happen to different people. We have only to deal with our own difficulties and let others deal with theirs.

Mentally Prepare Yourself to Heal

To heal yourself, acknowledge first that you have a condition that is not a normal part of a woman's lot. You can change your condition. The change you make may be small or large, but in either case it will be for the better. Some women will find that the changes are not drastic because they are already doing some of the things suggested in the self-help program. For others, the lifestyle changes will be radical.

Any self-help program — whether it concerns dieting, or giving up smoking, or something else — takes self-discipline. Not everyone can find it. Take a little time before starting the program to gather your strength and determination.

Affirmations

An affirmation is a positive statement said every day. It can be general, as in "I am free and happy," and can focus on what is happening now.

Or it can address aims for the future, as in "Today I will take one step closer to total well-being." Because it's not good to concentrate on your symptoms, it may not be a good idea to focus on endometriosis, as in "Today I will feel no pain." Instead, use your affirmations to focus on the good things that you experience, or want to experience, in your life.

The much-discussed healing power of prayer shows there are mysterious energies available. Instead of focusing on your endometriosis, perhaps direct your positive energy in ways that support the program, such as "Help my body to help itself," or "Give me strength while overcoming this health challenge," or "Help me to change my attitude toward my body."

Learn the Program

Learn how the self-help program works by reading through it a couple of times (see chapter 7). Collect the materials that you will need.

Find Emotional Support

Endometriosis is a difficult condition, not only because of the pain and other physical symptoms, but also because it may affect your self-image and self-esteem, your emotions, your sexuality, your fertility, your primary relationship, and even, sometimes, your ability to work. With luck, you have an understanding family and communicative health-care providers. If you belong to an endometriosis support group, you know other sufferers who can commiserate or celebrate with you. If you do not belong to a group, now might be a good time to find one. When you go through any self-help program, it helps to have emotional support. Identify a few key people, let them know what you are going to do, and ask if they will be on the end of the phone when you need to talk.

Get an Endo-Buddy

Your emotional support package could include an endo-buddy, someone else who has endometriosis and who will be more than interested in your progress. Ideally this will be someone who is, like you, interested in alternative approaches to the condition.

The self-help program will take several months. After a while, you will know which treatment strands are having the desired effect, and you can begin to design your own treatment. Keep a brief diary, noting your feelings, difficulties, and amusing moments (and there will be some). Share it all with your endo-buddy.

Take Time Out to Reflect

It may take you a day to reflect on the value of adopting this self-help program, or it may take a week, or months. Take as much time as you want — there's no need to rush into it. When you start the program, make sure you notice what's going on in your body. Make some "me" time. It can be whenever you like, but at least once a day shut the door, be still, be quiet, and listen to what your body has to tell you. Just take twenty minutes a day. Lie down and close your eyes, or sit up and stare into space. Take a walk or meditate. Wherever you spend your twenty minutes, listen to your body and notice how it's feeling. Some people call this centering, but primarily it's a matter of stopping still enough, long enough, to find yourself. If you can't help thinking about other people, then you've proven that you don't take enough time for yourself.

CHAPTER SIX

Detoxification

Throughout this program, you'll find references to adopting a healthier lifestyle in terms of food and water, exercise, essential oils, herbs, supplements, and stress reduction. Diet, for example, is important because it affects the working of your liver, which needs to be able to effectively process waste and manufacture proteins, including cholesterol. Diet has a direct effect on hormones, and if food contains environmental pollutants, this may contribute to inflammation and, as a result, produce pain.

The liver is the largest organ in the body, weighing between two and five pounds. It sits in the upper right portion of the abdominal cavity regulating all manner of physical functions. As well as absorbing oxygen and nutrients from the blood, the liver helps break down drugs and various toxins, manufactures proteins, and regulates blood glucose. The liver transforms one material into another, more useful, one. Hormones, including estrogen, progesterone, and testosterone, for example, are derived from cholesterol. We get a small amount of cholesterol from food, but most is produced by the liver.

The liver can't perform well if it has to deal with toxins coming into the body. When you are on the endometriosis self-help program, you need your body to function as well as it can. We cut down on alcohol, for example, because the liver is highly sensitive to it. For every liver-related illness not caused by alcohol consumption, there are five that are.

There are three types of estrogen, and although they are produced in different places within the body, they all derive from cholesterol. The liver transforms estrogen into bile, a less damaging form, which then goes to the intestines and is excreted from the body in feces. If the liver and/or gut are not working well, this normal excretion process cannot occur, and the waste estrogen will continue to circulate in the body, possibly stimulating it into estrogenic responses. This is not helpful if there is already an estrogen overload.

The liver is the immune system's first line of defense, and in one way it acts like a sponge, absorbing many of the dioxins, xenoestrogens, and other damaging chemicals that find their way into dairy products, meat, and fish. For the liver to be able to deal with these toxins, it must be strong and healthy, and diet can help. Increasing the amount of certain vegetables you eat, such as onions, garlic, and leeks, benefits good liver function by strengthening the liver's enzymes; also, pineapple can act as a good liver cleanser. The element magnesium encourages the activity of the enzyme glucuronyl transferase. This is one of the enzymes involved in hepatic glucuronidation — a chemical reaction in which hormones and toxins are linked by a water-soluble substance that inactivates the unwanted toxins and aids the elimination processes of urination and defecation. This linking process is known as "conjugation."

There are two types of cholesterol: the "good" high-density lipoproteins (HDL), the production of which diminishes after menopause, and the "bad" low-density lipoproteins (LDL), which can clog arteries. The vitamin B_3 (niacin) is said to draw LDL from the lining of the arteries and, as it lowers cholesterol, reduces the amount of estrogen in the body. The inositol-bound niacin supplements, inositol hexanicotinate, are preferable because this form isn't accompanied by flushing of the skin or gastrointestinal disturbance. Do not take niacin if you are trying to get pregnant.

Several herbs are known to have a beneficial effect on liver function, in particular milk thistle (see page 110). Artichoke leaf is said to reduce the degenerative effect of fat in the liver, and the culinary herb turmeric is an excellent antioxidant.

While detoxifying your body, it's essential to drink only water — if possible, spring water bottled in glass, not tap water. Eat organically grown food whenever possible. Reduce your use of strong hot spices, such as chili pepper and curries, and cut out all meat and salt. Eat mainly brown rice, fruit, and vegetables.

The liver does a good job of conjugating estrogens and excreting them in the bile. To exit the body, however, they have to pass through the gut, where they encounter bacteria. Some intestinal bacteria produce an enzyme called beta-glucuronidase which deconjugates estrogens, making them free to reenter the body instead of leaving in the feces. As this aggravates endometriosis, make sure the intestinal flora stays in balance by taking a daily probiotics supplement.

If the estrogens get through the gut, they have to come into contact with fiber — which they can attach to, and get excreted with. This is one reason why it is important to have fiber in the diet.

The overall aim of detoxification is to dislodge impurities from the body's tissues and eliminate them from the body by the usual means. It's a dynamic process, and this is not the time to overload the liver with fats, alcohol, nicotine, or stress.

CHAPTER SEVEN

The Endometriosis
Natural Treatment Program

The program outlined here has been used successfully over a period of fifteen years by many women attending a private clinic in the United Kingdom. This is the first time that the program has been made available to a wider group of women. Those women who completed the program all found that their symptoms diminished in varying degrees, and some women found it possible to conceive and became pregnant. To a large extent, the degree of a woman's success with this program depends on the degree of her commitment.

Many women will find diet or lifestyle suggestions here that they're already using, while others will have to consider a profound change in lifestyle. Some women reading this will follow all the recommendations, and others will follow a few. Each woman must choose for herself which route to take. As noted earlier, you can follow this program while continuing treatment by your physician.

Like all forms of treatment, this self-help program will suit some women, but not all. Some may prefer to use other treatments, such as acupuncture, herbalism, or homeopathy; information on these methods appears in a later chapter. Women who choose to follow those routes may nevertheless find strands of this program helpful.

ASSESSING AND DEALING
WITH OTHER HEALTH PROBLEMS

There are two types of health problems: those with symptoms we notice and can treat, and those known as "asymptomatic" (without symptoms). The term *asymptomatic* is somewhat misleading, because some of the conditions labeled this way do lead to symptoms; it's just that those symptoms are often misdiagnosed. For example, chlamydia, which is described as "asymptomatic," can produce symptoms such as pelvic pain, painful bowel movements, fever, and, if the infection spreads to the uterus, heavier and more painful periods. If an affected woman has not been specifically tested for *Chlamydia trachomatis*, the organism responsible for this infection, she or her physician may think she has pelvic inflammatory disease (PID), dysmenorrhea, or even endometriosis.

It is vital for any woman who thinks she has endometriosis, but who has not had a laparoscopy to confirm the diagnosis, to be tested for chlamydia. This organism is extremely common, and increasingly so. In the United States, one million women a year are treated for chlamydia, and a quarter of them are hospitalized. Untreated chlamydia develops into PID in 40 percent of cases and is one of the most common causes of female infertility.

Chlamydia often goes undetected because it is stigmatized as a sexually transmitted disease. In many countries such diseases are tested for only in special clinics, not by general physicians. Since many women do not attend the clinics, those with chlamydia remain untested and undiagnosed, and their condition gets worse by the day.

Other sexually transmitted organisms include *Ureaplasma urealyticum* and *Ureaplasma parvum*, known collectively as ureaplasma infections or "the genital mycoplasmas." These organisms — the mycoplasmas — are unusual because they have no cell walls and are exceedingly small, even in terms of microorganisms. For this reason, it takes highly specialized techniques to identify them, and simply getting them to a lab for testing requires exceptional care. Few physicians

3

routinely test for ureaplasma species, even though these microorganisms have been implicated in many diverse conditions, including pelvic inflammatory disease and endometriosis.

In the United States, studies have shown that 40 to 80 percent of sexually active women showing no signs of infection are actually carrying the ureaplasma species in the cervicovaginal area. These findings have huge implications for female reproductive health. Because the infection can be transmitted from mother to baby, it also has serious implications for infant health.

As knowledge about the ureaplasma species becomes more widespread and the facilities to test for it become more common, many previously mysterious but persistent health problems may be easier to treat with appropriate medications. But do not wait to be tested, because if you are indeed carrying this mycoplasma, your symptoms (which are probably now being blamed on something else, or on some mysterious unknown cause, or even on your imagination) will not go away unless treated.

Another health issue often overlooked is intestinal parasites. Although we worm our pets regularly, few people think they themselves could have worms, flukes, or other small creatures hitching a ride in their intestines or liver. Most of the time, parasites don't cause any immediate, visible problem, but they produce waste products and create toxins. It is not only international travelers who must consider this risk: it has been shown that the water supplies in many developed countries carry parasites. It is sensible to occasionally have an intestinal cleanse or colonic irrigation and an herbal liver cleanse to rid yourself of unwelcome visitors.

DIET: CHANGING TO ORGANIC AND UNPROCESSED FOODS

How much you'll have to change your diet depends entirely on what you eat now. If you eat only organically grown foods, and no processed foods, you could probably skip to the next section. If you find you

THE NATURAL TREATMENT PROGRAM

must make many changes in your diet, just do the best you can. What follows is an ideal eating plan — and we know that the ideal is not always possible in reality.

The endometriosis eating plan has nothing to do with fatness or thinness, nothing to do with weight. The diet is about reducing our intake of toxins — synthetic chemicals used in growing fruit and vegetables, and an array of antibiotics, hormones, and even metals injected into animals grown for meat. A 2002 report by the United Kingdom's Pesticide Safety Directorate showed that 43 percent of fruit and vegetables sold by British supermarkets contained chemical residues (up from 39 percent in 2001). This is despite the fact that certain supermarkets tell their suppliers not to use known problem chemicals. One well-known store chain forbade the use of the hormone-disrupter carbendazim, and yet this pesticide still turned up in its fresh apples, grapes, peaches, and cucumbers, among other produce items. If even the supermarkets don't know what is in these products, how can we? This is why you should — as far as you can — switch to organic.

If you must eat red meat, consume it no more frequently than once a week. Avoid all processed meats. Fresh chicken and fish are fine, but avoid shellfish and farmed fish. Dairy is out completely — no milk, yogurt, cottage cheese, goat milk products, or any other kind of manufactured milk product. Also, eat no cheese of any kind — including cheese for vegetarians, which is highly processed. Eat no wheat, wheat products, or soy products, including soymilk. Instead try all things made of oats, rice, quinoa, corn, and other grains. Help yourself to loads of fruit and vegetables — including those with starch, as they are good carbohydrates. Garlic and onions reduce inflammation, as does pineapple. Eggs are fine; legumes such as peas, lentils, and most beans are good.

Some food products, such as corn, are in some countries likely to be genetically modified (GM). There is a huge ongoing argument about GM food manufacturing processes, and until enough time has passed to ensure there are no unforeseen health repercussions, it may be better to err on the side of caution. Some GM seeds are grown in organic conditions, so look for labeling saying that a product is both "organic" and "non-GM."

Drink at least eight large glasses of still mineral water a day in addition to any other liquids. Avoid sodas (fizzy drinks), coffee, black tea (English breakfast, Earl Grey, Darjeeling, etc.), and hot chocolate, and instead stock up on a wide variety of fruit teas and herb teas. Green tea is acceptable in moderation, but with no milk or cream. Start making your own juices and smoothies as well. Water is essential to life, and dehydration is a common problem. Thirst is often mistaken for hunger, so have a glass of water instead of eating when you feel a little hungry.

Buy organic vegetable oils and vinegars, and make your own dressings. As noted, salt should be avoided at this time, but use as many herbs as you like in salads and when cooking. If you have a sweet tooth and crave sugar, use honey instead of sugar. You can eat nuts, so long as they are not roasted or salted. You can have raisins provided they're not covered in mineral oil, which is used to make them shiny and separate from each other. Dried fruit is often heavily processed, sometimes using dioxins, which have been implicated in the development of endometriosis. Seeds are great to munch on; try pumpkin or sunflower.

Garlic is not to everyone's taste, but it is high in antioxidants. It is also said to boost the immune system, reduce blood pressure, prevent blood clots, and bring glucose and serum levels down. Tests have shown the antibacterial properties of garlic, as well as of clove, cinnamon, orange, oregano, and sage. When you have a viral infection, it may be helpful to add oregano to the dinner pot, and cinnamon to the dessert. If you have physical problems to do with fungi or molds, thyme and oregano are the herbs of choice.

In essence, the endometriosis diet goes back to basics. Prepackaged ready-to-eat meals contain hidden additives and are off the menu, as is everything in cans. Wherever possible, get basic ingredients and cook them into delicious meals. Buy a few vegetarian cookbooks to get ideas. Because raw vegetables are said to be far more nutrient-rich than cooked ones, have uncooked vegetables as often as possible. This is easy to do if you make interesting salads prepared with a variety of raw vegetables.

Before starting the self-help program, spend a week writing down what you actually eat. The idea is to identify food groups that you overconsume. Overconsumption of a particular type of food could indicate an intolerance to it. Perversely, people often find themselves attracted to foods their bodies have difficulty tolerating.

Write down every single thing you eat or drink. Choose a week that is pretty normal, with no big celebrations or holidays, when everybody tends to indulge. If you dine out regularly, include that meal in your weekly record, noting whether it was Indian, Thai, Italian, or another type. Chinese food often contains monosodium glutamate, which women with endometriosis should avoid.

At the end of the week, add up the total portion units you have eaten in the following food groups:

- Wheat
- Dairy
- Fruit and vegetables
- Protein

It is remarkable how unhealthfully people eat, even when they think they have a healthy diet. The following diets are examples of weekly eating habits typical in many households (the predominant items are marked with an asterisk). Although people's weekend eating is often healthier, since there is more time to prepare food, they still consume their predominant food.

For example, in a typical week, Diet 1 incorporates a predominance of wheat:

Breakfast: Wheat cereal*; or toast,* bagel,* muffin,* or pastry*;
      tea or coffee

Midmorning: Cookies,* cake,* or pastry*; soda, tea, or coffee
Lunch: Sandwich,* hamburger,* or noodles*; soda
Midafternoon: Cookies,* cake,* or pastry*; soda, tea, or coffee
Evening meal: Pasta,* pasta sauce (with thickening agent*), garlic bread,* salad, dessert
Snacks: Cheese with crackers*; cookies* or bagels*; hot dog*; hamburger*

In a typical week, Diet 2 incorporates a predominance of dairy products (marked with asterisks):

Breakfast: Cereal with milk*; toast; glass of milk* or tea or coffee with milk*
Midmorning: Yogurt* or smoothie*
Lunch: Cheese* sandwich, ice cream,* coffee with cream*
Midafternoon: Tea or coffee with milk,* cake with cream filling* or cheese*-flavored snack
Evening meal: Macaroni and cheese,* pizza,* or pasta with cheese sauce*; glass of milk*
Snacks: Cheese* and bread; or yogurt,* ice cream,* milkshake,* or milk chocolate*

We've all heard about "a balanced diet," and this is what we're aiming for in the program. When you look at your weekly intake of food (and no cheating — don't identify a slice of gherkin on your hamburger as a serving of vegetable!), see if there is one type of food predominating. Unless it is fruit or vegetables, in the future eat only one portion of the predominant food group per day. If you feel you can't live without eating more of it, consider this: you may be sensitive to or intolerant of that food group or an ingredient contained in it. As noted earlier, we tend to crave the substances our bodies are sensitive to.

If this sounds like you, and you suffer bloating, hunger pains after eating, or any bowel disorder, take the prominent food out of your diet completely. You may suffer from withdrawal symptoms at first, but after a week you may notice an improvement in your well-being.

If indeed your body is intolerant to the predominant food, this will most likely become clear within four weeks.

If, on the other hand, you experience no change in your symptoms, most likely you are not intolerant to that food. If this is the case, slowly reintroduce it, one portion per day, but try to balance it better with other food groups this time.

AVOIDING TAP WATER AND WATER IN PLASTIC BOTTLES

Nothing is more basic than water or as precious. Water sustains all life. In fact, the average human body is at least 60 percent water. But we no longer gather our drinking water into our hands from a sparkling spring. We draw it from a tap or bring it home in a bottle. What are we drinking? Do we know? And what are we bathing in? Increasingly, the quality of tap water in the industrialized world is a cause for concern, for a variety of reasons.

The most obvious issue is biocides — that is, pesticides, herbicides, fungicides, and others. This includes not only those applied in recent years but also residues of those used a decade and more ago and still persisting in underground sources of water and elsewhere. The fluoridation of water has caused a great deal of debate. Apparently water utilities do not use the naturally occurring, nontoxic form of fluoride, calcium fluoride, in their treatment plants but instead add sodium fluoride and fluorosalicic acid, neither of which is found in nature. These compounds are added to water in some areas despite the fact that they are industrial by-products and so toxic that they are also used in rat poison and insecticides.

Another common, but worrying, addition to water is chlorine. When lying in a bath of chlorinated water, the body absorbs as much chlorine as it would from drinking eight pints of chlorinated water, according to one report. Some commentators say showers could be worse, because when the chlorine in the water hits the floor of the cubicle it releases chlorine gas, which is poisonous.

Among other things, the goal of water treatment is to eliminate cloudiness, kill bacteria, and adjust the pH balance — in other words, make it safe for humans to drink. To achieve this, a wide variety of substances are added, such as aluminum sulfate, phosphates, soda ash, lime, and carbon. Moreover, other substances have found their way into the water table — the fertilizers and pesticides applied on the land, for example, and chemicals in industrial waste. Another cause for uneasiness is radium, which has been detected in some sources of public water in the United States and has been said to be implicated in the increased incidence of leukemia and other cancers.

Water packaging is also a concern, because plastic bottles are often made of chemicals (xenoestrogens) that mimic the action of estrogen, and these may leach into the water. Imagine that — you thought you were drinking a glassful of water and it turns out to be hormone replacement therapy!

Having said all this, let me stress the point that it's extremely important to drink plenty of water. We need water to digest food, metabolize nutrients, and flush out our metabolic waste. Without water, lactic acid and acid urea cannot be dissolved and eliminated from the body by the kidneys. Water is needed for efficient blood flow, which in turn brings oxygen and food to the cells. But where can we get the best possible water? An entire industry has opened up to provide the answer. Not only can you buy a huge variety of designer mineral waters in every supermarket, but you can also purchase equipment to purify water at home through such methods as steam distillation, reverse osmosis, and activated alumina filtration. Filtration systems for the entire home are available, as are kitchen, bath, and shower filters.

No filtration system can remove *all* of the contaminants in tap water, so it is important for you to look into the options available to you, research the subject of water in your area, and make a decision about what steps you must take to ensure a supply of pure water — both to drink and to bathe in. Several useful water information sites

THE NATURAL TREATMENT PROGRAM

are available on the Web, and in the United States specific local information can be obtained through the Water Quality Association based in Lisle, Illinois. Many private companies test water quality. Look after your water, and your water will look after you.

EXERCISE

The exercise regime for women with endometriosis is not about losing weight. Nonetheless, it is worth bearing in mind that, because estrogen is thought to be stored in fat, overweight women may be carrying around extra estrogen with their extra weight. This is important because endometriosis is thought to be exacerbated by an excess of estrogen in the body.

Exercise is important because it seems to play a part in reducing pain, perhaps by making the adhesions less rigid. Movement certainly makes the body stronger and more energized. Any type of exercise is good, so long as it's gentle, not the tough, cardiovascular type. Even just dancing around the room to your favorite music is exercise, but it must be done on a regular basis.

It's well known that excessive exercise reduces the number of menstrual cycles some women experience, even delaying the onset of puberty in gymnasts, for example. This demonstrates a direct relationship between exercise and the body's production of hormones. But hormone disruptions are likely to occur in many subtle ways we are not yet entirely aware of — as a result of both too much exercise and too little. We all know the body requires a certain amount of exercise to keep it functioning at its best — and this includes the endocrine system, or hormones. It's thought that regular, gentle exercise regulates hormone activity and helps prevent overproduction.

Too much exercise puts stress on the body and uses up valuable B vitamins and minerals, such as zinc and magnesium. But consider the benefits of regular gentle exercise: increased circulation, leading to improved function of organs and muscles, including those of the pelvic area; a stimulated lymphatic system, leading to a more effective immune system; and an improved digestive system, leading to better elimination. Interestingly, studies have shown that exercise causes both estrogen and cholesterol to be eliminated from the body by excretion. Exercise is known to improve the functioning of the thyroid gland, leading to better metabolism. It also helps keep the body's blood sugar in balance, and causes the release of endorphins — brain chemicals that have a positive effect on stress, anxiety, and depression. Regular exercise increases a sense of well-being. It is also said to lower the level of low-density lipoproteins (LDL), the bad cholesterol, while elevating high-density lipoproteins (HDL), the good cholesterol. And, while you might think exercise makes you tired, in fact it increases energy levels and endurance generally. Follow exercise regimes that put no strain on your internal organs.

Swimming is an excellent form of total body exercise for women with endometriosis, because the water supports your body while you make a wide range of movements using all your limbs, at your own pace. There is a downside, however: most pools are treated with chlorine, which is breathed in around the pool and absorbed through the skin when in contact with the water. According to the British Government's Committee on Toxicity, which assessed research carried out at Imperial College, London, in 2004, chlorine may harm pregnant women and their fetuses, possibly causing miscarriage, low birth weight, or stillbirth. This research seems to confirm work carried out in Norway and Canada that suggests a link between chlorine and higher rates of birth defects and bowel, kidney, and bladder cancer. Given these potential risks, if you choose to swim, it would be wise to seek out pools that use the minimum amount of chlorine, and avoid them on days when the chlorine is added. Better still, try to find a pool that uses alternative water-treatment methods that are more environmentally friendly. If you have your own pool, consider changing to less harmful water-treatment methods.

Brisk walking or gentle jogging are invigorating, if you are comfortable doing them. Dance is a good form of workout if it is free-form — where you are able to follow your own chosen movements, rather than following a set of sharp, predesigned movements determined by someone else (whose body may not be experiencing pain, as yours does). Feel free to join a salsa class, but keep the movements under your own control.

Certain exercise forms originating in Asia are ideal for endometriosis sufferers — tai chi, chi gong, and certain types of yoga, for example — and they can be practiced at home or in a class. If you have a teacher, inform this person of your condition and he or she will be able to adapt the movements to your requirements. These gentle Eastern movement systems are good not only for the body but also for the mind and spirit. You'll feel invigorated but calm.

BODY BRUSHING

Body brushing is included in the endometriosis treatment program because it's an excellent way to detoxify the body. It is a technique designed to stimulate the flow of lymph. Some women will prefer to omit this section of the treatment program because they believe the hypothesis that endometriosis is caused by endometrial cells from the uterus being transported through lymph to distant parts of the body. However, if endometrial cells could be transported in this way (and there is no evidence for it), many more women — perhaps all women — would have endometrial tissue showing up all over their bodies. Clearly, this is not the case. Also, as exercise increases the flow of lymph, adherents of the "lymphatic flow theory" might say that the more women exercise, the more likely it is that endometrial cells from their uterus will become misplaced elsewhere. If this were the case, the entire exercise industry would have come to a halt long ago, and women would be confined to their couches. But you must make your own informed choice on this issue. Please refer to pages 26–27.

THE LYMPHATIC SYSTEM

Like the blood circulatory system, the lymphatic system is a bodywide transportation system. It has often been described as resembling a string of pearls, with the pearls being lymph nodes. The tiny, delicate vessels transport a milky fluid known as lymph. This is absorbed from the cells of body tissues, into which it leaks through the walls of blood capillaries. There is a constant back-and-forth movement as blood plasma is leaked into the cells, then absorbed into the lymph, where it is cleaned in the nodules, and then returned to the blood. Just under four and a half gallons of liquid is exchanged each day. The lymph both cleanses tissues in this way and provides cells with oxygen and nutrients.

The lymphatic system is directed by the thymus gland, located behind the breastbone. It has no pumping station, such as the heart, which pumps blood; instead the lymphatic system is driven by the natural movements of the body. The less you exercise, the lower the lymphatic flow, and the less cleansing can take place. The lymph system, along with the spleen and bone marrow, produces leukocytes, which in turn produce antibodies that attack invading microorganisms.

The "pearls" of the lymphatic system, the nodules, are where the cleansing action takes place. If there is an infection in the body, the nodules become enlarged as they battle to control the invading microbes. These enlarged nodules are the "swollen glands" that so often accompany bacterial and viral infections.

Body brushing is said to help accomplish the following:

- stimulate the flow of lymph
- stimulate the flow of connective tissue fluid

- stimulate the flow of blood, increasing oxygenation and tissue health
- remove cell waste or debris from the connective tissue
- encourage the functioning of the lymphatic defense system
- balance the nervous system
- clear dead skin cells from the surface of the skin so that products are absorbed more readily

Use a natural bristle brush, and brush your skin in the direction of the flow of the body's lymphatic system. The hand-held variety of brush is easier to control. Brush your body in the morning, or before showering. It can feel a bit odd at first, but after a while you'll appreciate the invigoration and will soon wonder how you ever got along without it. The effects on blood circulation and the skin are secondary and have no relevance to the technique used.

Contraindications

There are circumstances in which stimulating lymph flow is not advised. In particular, because the job of the nodules is to trap and fight the microorganisms that cause infections, you do not want to stimulate the lymph flow and cause those organisms to be flushed out of the nodules while they are still active. Do not, therefore, brush your body while you have an acute infection. If you have had tuberculosis (TB) in the past, it may not be advisable to body-brush; it has been said that TB bacilli may be trapped in the nodules and become activated.

You should not brush your body if you have had a recent thrombosis, as there may be a risk of embolism, or if you have heart edema, an insufficiency of the right side of the heart. During menstruation, omit step 5 in the brushing technique outlined below. Omit steps 7 and 8 in the brushing technique if you have asthma.

The Body-Brushing Technique

In addition to the main vessels of the lymphatic system, there are tiny capillaries known as "initial lymph vessels," which together make up an extremely fine and delicate system. If you think of the blood circulatory system as coarsely woven wool, then the lymphatic system is like silk. With body brushing, the aim is not to stimulate the flow of blood by using rough strokes. Instead, it is important to use only delicate and light brushstrokes. Heavy brushstrokes only press blood from one tissue to another and can actually constrict lymph vessels, as if you were pressing on a garden hose — nothing can get through.

Start your brushstrokes on the front of the body, then move on to the back of the body; in each area of the body, start with brushstrokes on the left side before moving to the right. All the movements should be light and gentle. Brush each section three to four times before moving on to the next section of the body.

1. Left foot: brush the sole of the left foot toward the heel. Then brush the top of the foot from toes to ankle.
2. Left leg: brush up the front of the lower left leg in long vertical strokes, ankle to knee, then brush the back of the lower leg, Achilles tendon to back of knee. Brush the front of the upper leg, from the knee to the top of the thigh, then the back of the upper leg, from the back of the knee to the buttock.
3. Right foot and leg: repeat steps 1 and 2 on the right side.
4. Pelvis-hip area: brush around the left hip, from back to front. Make several large vertical sweeps, working upward from the bottom panty line until you reach the pelvic bone. Repeat on the right side.
5. Waist: brush from the center of your back, around the waist toward the front of your body, then downward toward, but not as far as, the groin. Repeat on the other side.
6. Abdomen: follow a horseshoe shape, starting on the lower right side, traveling up in a vertical line, then left across the diaphragm, and down the left side of the abdomen in a straight line. Then imagine a large clock shape on your belly, and brush each five-minute section of that clock — inward toward the navel, using short strokes.

7. Arms: brush in long strokes up the inside and outside of the left arm to the armpit. Repeat on the right arm.
8. Upper chest area (above the breasts) and shoulders: brush inward in short strokes toward the sternum (the bone in the center of the upper chest). Include the shoulders. Do this on the right side first, and then the left.

ESSENTIAL OILS

Essential oils offer a multifaceted approach to endometriosis. Each essential oil can perform a variety of functions at the same time. This is possible because essential oils could contain up to several hundred components, each of which may have a particular therapeutic action. One of the most important essential oils for treating endometriosis is geranium (*Pelargonium graveolens*). The sidebar "Geranium (*Pelargonium graveolens*)" lists some of geranium's therapeutic properties and how they can affect endometriosis.

As we have seen in the previous chapters, the cause of endometriosis is unknown and many theories about the cause have been put forward. When using essential oils, we do not need to know which of the proposed theories is correct, because we don't take a single approach. We move forward on all fronts at the same time.

The key is being able to choose the right essential oils to use. For example, lavender oil is thought to affect the liver by slowing down its release of glucose, and research has shown that helichrysum, also known as Italian everlasting, "jump-starts" the functioning of the liver. It is also thought to be anti-inflammatory, anticoagulant, regenerative, and analgesic.

Particularly Valuable Essential Oils for Endometriosis

According to many endometriosis specialists, the pain results from an inflammatory reaction in the peritoneal area and does not correspond to the number of the endometriosis implants or growths or the extent of the resulting scar tissue. If this is so, anti-inflammatory

GERANIUM (*Pelargonium graveolens*)

Therapeutic Properties	Possible Effects on Endometriosis
Antispasmodic	Calms contractions of uterus
Anti-inflammatory	Reduces inflammation and pain
Stimulates lymphatic system	Helps clear body of toxins
Stimulates liver and pancreas	Allows production of vital enzymes and cholesterol
Antifungal, antiyeast	May control *Candida albicans* and other yeasts and fungi
Antibacterial	May control unwanted bacterial activity without affecting intestinal flora
Antiseptic	Controls infection
Homeostatic	Stops bleeding
Anticoagulant	Helps prevent blood clots
Calms sympathetic and parasympathetic systems	Balances the nervous system
Antidepressant	Assists in alleviating depression

essential oils, such as Italian everlasting (*Helichrysum angustifolium*), chamomile German (*Matricaria recutita*), chamomile Roman (*Anthemis nobilis*), lavender (*Lavandula angustifolia*), eucalyptus radiata (*Eucalyptus radiata*), and yarrow (*Achillea millefolium*), are helpful.

The antispasmodics, such as marjoram (*Origanum marjorana*), clary sage (*Salvia sclarea*), chamomile Roman, and rose otto (*Rosa damascena*), are also valuable in controlling the uterine spasms that may accompany endometriosis. Rose is also considered to be antiseptic, antibacterial, and relaxing, and is a mild analgesic.

If bloating is a problem, a diuretic such as juniper (*Juniperus communis*) might be recommended. If the lymph flow is slow, a decongestant for veins and lymph, such as cypress (*Cupressus sempervirens*), will be more appropriate. All women appreciate the relaxing effect of neroli (*Citrus aurantium*) essential oil and the calming and balancing effect of bergamot (*Citrus aurantium* ssp. *bergamia*). This is the other advantage of essential oils — they have a positive effect on the emotions.

Useful Functions of Certain Essential Oils in the Control of Endometriosis

Balancing Hormones

It is helpful to distinguish between the different ways hormones can be regulated:

- The most obvious way is to add hormones to the body, for example, through birth control pills or hormone replacement therapy (HRT); the hormones consumed in tablet form increase the amount of those hormones circulating around the body.
- A second way to regulate hormones is through diet and lifestyle, because the liver plays such an important role in hormone manufacture, as does the thyroid.
- Another way to regulate hormones is to introduce a phyto-hormone that binds with the hormone receptor and blocks the uptake and response of that hormone.

Essential oils are likely to work in the third way, blocking the hormone receptor and preventing overload. They do this as phytoestrogens, plant chemicals that function as hormones in the body.

In the *Journal of Biological Chemistry*, scientist Jinping An and colleagues published an article that begins: "Estrogens used in hormone replacement therapy regimes may increase the risk of developing breast cancer. Paradoxically, high consumption of plant-derived phytoestrogens, particularly soybean isoflavones, is associated with a low incidence of breast cancer." It concludes: "Phytoestrogens may act as natural selective estrogen receptor modulators" (2001). These SERMs, as they are known, block certain hormone receptors, reducing the uptake of that particular hormone. Although they behave like estrogen, phytoestrogens seem to reduce the amount of estrogen actually used by the body.

There are two estrogen receptors on cells, known as ER-α (estrogen receptor alpha) and ER-ß (estrogen receptor beta). According to researchers Julie Hall and Kenneth Korach (2002), these receptors respond differently to xenoestrogens, the hormone-disrupting chemicals that come into the body in a variety of ways.

THE THREE ESTROGENS

The estrogenic potency of estradiol is twelve times that of estrone and eighty times that of estriol.

It's worth remembering that we're always learning new things about hormones and about other aspects of physiology we thought were already fully understood. In May 2003 researchers Roger Pierson and his associates showed the results of the ovarian follicle movement and ovulation of fifty women tested every day for a month by transvaginal ultrasonography. These researchers found that follicles in the ovary may develop not just once a month but two or three times. This finding, which confirms much other evidence gathered previously, including veterinary evidence, has huge implications for contraceptive pill manufacture, in vitro fertilization, and childbirth procedures.

The researchers say that much more work must be done before they can accurately measure the luteinizing hormones and follicle-stimulating hormones produced by women over the course of a month. In other words, we really can't guarantee that we can accurately predict their ebb and flow during the menstrual cycle. It turns out we didn't know as much as we thought we did — and that's how science is: it moves on.

Human beings have ingested or otherwise used phytoestrogens since time began. Perhaps they ate the plant material, made it into drinks, or sprinkled it on other foods. They made herbal inhalants and breathed them in. They made lotions and potions and rubbed them on their bodies. Plants are used in a thousand ways by human beings, and all these ways can get plant phytohormones into the body. Phytohormones are part of the environment — we smell a rose in the garden, or we crush a geranium leaf in our fingers and inhale the sweet aroma. Our bodies are used to these things, and we have learned over millennia that they do us no harm. We've gained common sense based on years of observation and knowledge.

Stimulating Liver Function

The liver is not a glamorous organ, and generally we don't hear much about it, but the liver is extremely important in all medical conditions and is vital to life itself. For a woman with endometriosis, the liver is particularly important because it creates the cholesterol that is transformed into hormones — including estrogen, progesterone, and testosterone. This is achieved in several biochemical steps by the actions of specialist enzymes.

When the liver is functioning well, it keeps hormone production at the optimal levels. When the liver is overloaded with toxins, many apparently unrelated organs and body systems fail to work correctly.

Oxygenation

Certain essential oils stimulate the blood to flow more easily, increasing the distribution of oxygen and leading to tissue regeneration and healing. This oxygenation also helps the process of removing toxins from the body.

Encouraging Immune System Function

Good lymphatic flow supports the immune system, which contains countless mobile cells, such as macrophages, that fight to eliminate unwanted substances from the body. They keep us internally clean and unharmed by invading microorganisms, misplaced cells, and environmental toxins. Some essential oils appear to stimulate the lymphatic system, encouraging it to work efficiently.

Antimicrobial

There is a wide variety of essential oils, and they vary in their ability to challenge bacteria, viruses, fungi, and mycoplasmas. Two of the most impressive, as shown in laboratory tests, are oregano (*Origanum vulgare*) and thyme (*Thymus vulgaris*), but the majority of essential oils have some antimicrobial qualities.

Other essential oils have shown little antimicrobial effect in the laboratory but in practice do show an ability to prevent the proliferation of bacteria. This effect is thought to be a result of the essential oil boosting the immune system — which then more efficiently destroys the bacteria.

Stomach ulcers were thought to be the result of an acid-alkaline imbalance — until 1983, when it was discovered that the bacterium *Helicobacter pylori* was more likely the cause. Treatment changed overnight and became more effective. It now seems that a wide range of conditions have potential links to a bacterial cause, including certain types of asthma, arthritis, cancer, mental disorders, multiple sclerosis, and heart disease. Another problem related to bacteria is that types that are normally harmless can become misplaced — the killers meningitis and necrotizing fasciitis, for example, are caused by bacteria getting out of control. Harmless in one body location, some bacteria become lethal in another location, especially the bloodstream. In some cases, this may be due to an injury, but in many more people it occurs for reasons as yet unknown.

Although endometriosis has never been associated with a bacterium (of which there are around five thousand types identified so far) or virus (five thousand types), it is an enigmatic and mysterious disease, and we have to keep our minds open when considering possible causes. The only microorganisms that have been linked so far to endometriosis are the mycoplasmas, the smallest of organisms; sixteen of these have been found in humans. The two of particular interest to us are ureaplasmas. The study of these organisms is still relatively new, and the link to endometriosis untested, and so currently no treatments for endometriosis exist that take ureaplasmas as its cause. However, if ever such a link is found, essential oils will be standing by ready to fight the fight.

Bacteria are not all bad. In fact, without them we would rot and die. They convert the food we eat into vitamins and energy, they process our waste, clean our internal water, and make amino acids from nitrogen in the air. What makes essential oils so good at dealing with the complex life of bacteria and other microorganisms is that they are natural products that the human body has adapted to. Cinnamon (*Cinnamomum zeylanicum*), for example, is one of the most effective antimicrobials known, and human beings have been using it to spice up their food for as long as history can show. Experience has demonstrated that this aromatic spice is powerful enough to get rid of the bacteria that make us ill, without giving us side effects.

Antispasmodic

Choosing essential oils extracted from the correct, specific species of plant is important, a fact highlighted by the case of muscle spasm. There are hundreds of species of geranium plants around the world, and many are used in local folk medicine. In South Africa, local inhabitants use a geranium called *Pelargonium grossularioides* as an abortifacient because it is a spasmogenic and causes the uterus to contract. This effect has been confirmed by laboratory tests on rat uteruses. On the other hand, other types of geraniums do the opposite: they make smooth muscle tissue relax, such as in the uterus (they are "spasmolytic"). In this program we use *Pelargonium graveolens* or *Pelargonium odorantissimum*, both of which relax uterine muscle.

When choosing essential oils to treat endometriosis, it's important to know the exact species of plant your essential oil has been extracted from. Increasingly, reputable suppliers print the botanical (Latin) name of the species on the bottle. Always look for it when using essential oils for health reasons.

THE NATURAL TREATMENT PROGRAM

Analgesic

Anyone who has felt the relief of pure lavender oil (*Lavandula angustifolia*) on the pain of a burn or insect bite will tell you that essential oils can be analgesic. It may be hard to believe that the sweet-smelling lavender oil and rose otto oil (*Rosa damascena*), so often thought of as just perfumes, can also do the hard-hitting job of pain relief, but they can. This reminds us not to be fooled into thinking essential oils are weak simply because they smell divine.

It's always been one of the mysteries of endometriosis that, as noted earlier, some women with many implants can feel little pain, while some women with few implants can feel a great deal of pain. Some specialists have suggested this may be because certain women experience more inflammation in the affected areas than others. The most well-known anti-inflammatory essential oils are chamomile Roman (*Anthemis nobilis*), chamomile German (*Matricaria recutita*), and yarrow (*Achillea millefolium*). However, many other essential oils, such as lavender, have a anti-inflammatory effect.

Reducing Inflammation

Inflammation and pain go hand in hand. Eliminate inflammation, and pain tends to fade. Essential oils have been used for centuries to reduce inflammation, and a great deal of evidence exists for this aspect of their function.

Diuretic

Bloating can be the cause of a great deal of discomfort for women with endometriosis. Certain essential oils, such as cypress (*Cupressus sempervirens*) and juniper (*Juniperus communis*), can act as a natural diuretic, allowing the body to release fluid and lessen internal pressure of the tissues.

Relaxing

The relaxing properties of essential oils are one of their best-known aspects. Many people still think essential oils are only for relaxation. As with all essential oils, everything depends on choice — and while some essential oils are relaxing, bear in mind that others are stimulating. The relaxing or stimulating effect of various essential oils has been tested using brain imaging techniques for over a decade, and there is now little doubt that essential oils affect the psyche in many ways.

The Electrochemical Factor

Like all living beings, humans constantly undergo electrochemical processes. Our brains generate electrical energy, which passes through nerve fibers and activates muscles. The nerves of the muscles have a frequency that reaches as high as 250 Hz. That is a strong muscle reaction; less strong movement is driven by a lower frequency.

On a cellular level, we constantly experience a play between negative and positive charges. Cell membranes can have either a positive volt potential or a negative volt potential, and these determine whether positive ions will leave a cell, or enter it, and also whether negative ions will enter or leave.

Different neurotransmitters — chemical messengers used by the brain — have a wide range of effects on electrical signals. Not only do they make them fire, but they can inhibit them too. They can slow the electrical signal down or speed it up. Neurotransmitters can store energy and change the frequency of energy. They respond to our individual needs, which can be altered by our mood, diet, or health.

In the body as elsewhere, electricity is transmitted by electrons, and these come in two forms: left spin and right spin. This is a language the body understands and responds to. This is polarization, light-twisting properties, the negative/positive interplay at the basis of life. It is all part of the transformational dynamic that takes place all the time: cells building up, cells closing down — and being reformed as something else. Electricity catalyzes this process, being able to completely change matter — from solid to liquid, for example.

Essential oils have left-reflecting forms and right-reflecting forms. They come from plants, which, like all living things, contain liquid crystal — first discovered in 1888 in the extract of raw carrot. This dance between left and right enters into the constant dance of polarity in the human body, and it fits right in, not only chemically but electrically as well.

The human body is a great conductor of electricity because it's mostly water — estimates of the percentage of water vary between 60 and 90 percent. This is our medium, the electrical environment that essential oils enter into with such ease. These oils and we are part of the vibrating, oscillating dance of life, and if harmony can be achieved, changes are possible.

Using Essential Oils
for the Endometriosis Self-Help Program

Essential oils are a crucial element of the program. The key to success lies in choosing appropriate essential oils and using them as described here, preferably in all three methods recommended below. You will need to make or purchase several healing formulas. These are blends of several essential oils; whenever possible, purchase only those that have been derived from organically grown plants.

For the essential oil blends to be effective, it's important that the relative proportions of the essential oils are measured accurately. This can be done only if each drop added is the same size. Fortunately, suppliers tend to use the same type and size of dropper inserts in each of their bottles, so purchasing all the required essential oils from a single supplier will usually provide a solution to this potential problem. Alternatively, you can use droppers (pipettes) of your own, which can be bought at drug stores, pharmacies, or specialty stores. Remove the dropper inserts from the bottles, then use the pipette to measure the drops of essential oil. (See the sidebar "Skin Sensitivity Test" before using essential oils.)

Daily Essential Oil Methods

The methods for daily use of essential oils include the following:

- Sitz baths (once or twice a day)
- Hip and abdominal massage oil (once a day)
- Bath oils (once a day if possible)

SKIN SENSITIVITY TEST

Before using any essential oil or essential oil blend, carry out a skin sensitivity test. Smear a small amount of the oil in the crook of your arm and check it periodically over a twenty-four-hour period to see if you have an allergic reaction to that oil or to any ingredient in the blend.

Preparing Your Blends

To prepare the essential oil blends and massage oils presented in this chapter, you will need a set of metric measuring spoons or cylinders, preferably in stainless steel or glass, respectively. These are available for purchase online (type "metric measuring spoons and cylinders" into your favorite search engine) or in a pharmaceutical supply store. You will need spoons or cylinders that have the measurements in increments of 1 milliliter upward to 30 milliliters. Also, liquid over-the-counter medicines (such as cough syrups) are often sold with small measuring cups that have the measurements in milliliters — most pharmacists and drugstores have these available for sale.

You can either blend the essential oils each day or prepare a bigger volume of the blend for longer-term use. Whichever method you use, the blending method is the same: Put the drops of essential oil in a new, dry bottle and mix them together by replacing the lid, turning the bottle upside down a few times, then rolling the bottle vigorously between your hands. Label the bottle "Endometriosis (Sitz-Bath/Massage/or Bath) Blend," and add your name and the date. Leave the bottle to stand for twenty-four hours to allow the essential oils to combine before using.

SITZ BATHS

The sitz bath element of the endometriosis self-help treatment program is vital to its success. It would be ideal if you could follow all elements of the essential oil treatment strand, but if you cannot for any reason, and choose to do just one thing, this is it. If you are trying to get pregnant, the sitz bath element of the program is especially helpful.

A sitz bath is basically a small bath you lower your bottom into, so that the water covers just your rear end and your abdomen up to the navel. In the endometriosis sitz bath treatment, two baths are used — one hot, one cold.

For centuries sitz baths have been recommended in Europe by traditional healers such as herbalists and naturopaths. The sitz bath is a simple hydrotherapy method found in the natural healing traditions of Switzerland, Germany, Austria, France, Italy, Spain, and the eastern European countries. It's used for any type of disorder, disease, or inflammatory condition that affects the lower abdominal area of men and women. In women, this includes reproductive problems, such as those affecting the uterus, ovaries, and fallopian tubes, as well as pelvic inflammatory disease. This method is also used for other disorders, including digestive disorders such as constipation, and for hemorrhoids, anal fissures, lower back problems, and spasms or cramping of the lower limbs.

Contraindications

As this method involves alternating between hot and cold stimuli, it could bring about dramatic short-term changes in blood pressure. Therefore the sitz bath method should not be used if you have high blood pressure, deep vein thrombosis, arteriosclerosis, or any heart condition.

Key Elements of the Sitz Bath Treatment

- Ideally, have two sitz bath sessions per day — one in the morning, and one in the evening — as this seems to bring about a more rapid change than completing only one sitz bath session per day.

- Each session consists of alternate hot and cold sitz baths. You lower yourself into the hot water, then the cold water, and so on. One hot, plus one cold immersion constitutes one cycle. Do three to five cycles per session, depending on the severity of your case. Stay in each sitz bath for 2 minutes. The time required for three sitz bath cycles is 12 minutes (2 minutes each in hot and cold sitz baths = 4 minutes × 3 cycles).

- The water should cover the lower abdomen, upper thighs, and groin area. Ideally, the water will reach as high as your hips, but whether this happens depends on the equipment you use. Special sitz bath units are sometimes available through medical supply companies; alternatively use two baby baths, or two deep plastic basins large enough to sit in.

If you have a large bathtub, you might be able to fit two baby baths in it. If you can't fit two baby baths in your tub, use one baby bath and a large, deep plastic basin. If you do not have a bathtub, just place the baby baths or basins near each other on the bathroom floor.

Sitz baths may not be the most modern or convenient method, but they continue to be popular because they are so effective. The alternation between hot and cold water increases blood flow to the pelvis and abdominal area. As the muscles alternately contract with the cold and dilate with the heat, a unique healing stimulation takes place. Lymphatic flow is also increased, and congestion is removed from tissues. Inflammation, swelling, and bloating are reduced and tissue tone is improved. The specific essential oils used in these methods enhance the therapeutic process.

The Cold Sitz Bath

The cold sitz bath must contain very cold water. (After a few days, when you think you can tolerate it, add one or more ice cubes to the water to make it even colder.) Add to the cold water 10 milliliters

($^1/_3$ of a fluid ounce) of rose hydrolat or rose water. Rose hydrolat and rose water are mostly sold in units of 100 to 500 milliliters. You will need 600 milliliters (20 fluid ounces) per month. Buy organic if at all possible.

Hydrolat and rose water are by-products of essential oil production. Hydrolat is not diluted, as rose water often is. Both are watery and have a rose smell. These water-based products differ from pure essential oil of rose and should not be confused with it.

The Hot Sitz Bath

The pure essential oil blend (see the sidebar "Essential Endo Sitz Bath Blend") is used only in the hot sitz bath. The water for this sitz bath must be hot, but not uncomfortably so. Add 9 drops of the sitz bath blend of essential oils listed. Then swish the water around with your hand before sitting in it, so no oil globules remain on the surface to irritate the delicate mucous membrane of the genital area. Ensure that the water temperature is comfortable before lowering yourself in.

ESSENTIAL ENDO SITZ BATH BLEND

Geranium (*Pelargonium graveolens*)	4 drops
Rose otto (*Rosa damascena*)	20 drops
Cypress (*Cupressus sempervirens*)	8 drops
Nutmeg (*Myristica fragrans*)	40 drops
Clary sage (*Salvia sclarea*)	32 drops

Blend these oils together, then use 9 drops of the mixture for each hot sitz bath.

The mixture constitutes one week's supply, if using two sitz baths per day, with a little allowance for spillage. Do not be tempted to use more drops than recommended. In essential oil use, more is not necessarily better. In fact, sometimes less is best.

The Special Weekly Sitz Bath

On one day each week, do the sitz bath differently — use both baths at the same time, with your rear end in one and your feet in the other. As usual, fill one bath with cold water, and one with hot. Add the 10 milliliters of rose water or rose hydrolat to the cold water, and 9 drops of the Essential Endo Sitz Bath Blend to the hot water.

Start by lowering your rear end into the cold water, and let the water cover your lower abdomen. Now put your feet into the hot water, and sit for 2 minutes. Then, change over so your rear goes in the hot water and your feet in the cold — again for 2 minutes. This alternation constitutes one cycle. Repeat the cycle three more times.

If you have severe menstrual cramps, this method will help ease the pain. In this case, stay with your rear end in the hot bath for 3 minutes, and sit in the cold water for only 1 minute, for two or three cycles. If at any time you feel dizzy, nauseated, or faint, stop the treatment for that day. After the sitz bath, use the Low-Abdominal-Pain Synergy Blend for Hip Massage on page 97, up to 8 drops in 5 milliliters of vegetable oil (sometimes called "base" or "carrier" oil), rubbed over your abdomen.

EASY OPTION FOR THE SITZ BATH: THE ALTERNATIVE WAY

Not everyone will be able to carry out the sitz bath element of this program. Some may not be agile enough to move repeatedly between two sitz baths on the floor, or they may have only one baby bath to use as a sitz bath. Or they simply may want an easier option. Whatever the reason, there is an easy alternative to the usual sitz bath routine that forms such an important part of this self-help program. This option has a disadvantage: it is not as effective in helping you overcome endometriosis. It's a second-best option, but it's better than nothing. Remember, this can be substituted for the sitz bath portion of this program only; all other aspects of the program must be followed.

- Run a bath — hot, but not so hot that it is uncomfortable for you. Add 9 drops of the Essential Endo Sitz Bath Blend and swish it around.
- Relax in the bath for about 15 minutes, or less if you are feeling uncomfortable, adding more hot water as the bath cools. The heat will allow the vessels and capillaries of the circulation system to dilate and increase the flow of blood, bringing more oxygen to the organs.
- Lower your rear end in a cold sitz bath, to which you have added 10 milliliters of rose hydrolat or rose water.
- Stay in the cold sitz bath for 5 minutes, if you can.
- Do this routine every day.

THE HIP MASSAGE

Massage is a universally recognized way to release tension, ease pain, increase circulation, and bring oxygen to the massaged area. We use massage in the endometriosis self-help program not only for these reasons but also because it is a time-honored and effective way to deliver the active components of the essential oils into the body. In this program, a specific area is massaged — the hips — but if you are having a general, full body massage, you can take the endometriosis hip massage oil along and ask your therapist to use it as outlined here.

The daily hip massage takes only five minutes and is very easy. You may find it more convenient to do the hip massage after your evening sitz bath session.

ENDO HIP MASSAGE OIL BLEND

Dilute the following essential oils in 30 milliliters (1 fluid ounce) of almond or vegetable oil:

Clary sage (*Salvia sclarea*)	20 drops
Rose otto (*Rosa damascena*)	10 drops
Chamomile Roman (*Anthemis nobilis*)	4 drops
Geranium (*Pelargonium graveolens*)	20 drops
Lavender (*Lavandula angustifolia*)	16 drops

For each massage, use as much as required to cover the whole of the hip and abdominal area.

If you want, you can prepare larger amounts of undiluted essential oil in advance, ready for dilution later. Use the volumes and proportions shown below in the sidebar "Endo Hip Massage Oil Blend (Synergistic Blend)" to make 15 milliliters ($^1/_2$ fluid ounce) of the synergistic blend of essential oils.

ENDO HIP MASSAGE OIL BLEND (SYNERGISTIC BLEND)

Make a synergistic blend of essential oils using the following amounts:

Clary sage (*Salvia sclarea*)	3 milliliters
Rose otto (*Rosa damascena*)	3 milliliters
Chamomile Roman (*Anthemis nobilis*)	3 milliliters
Geranium (*Pelargonium graveolens*)	5 milliliters
Lavender (*Lavandula angustifolia*)	1 milliliter

When required, dilute the essential oil blend in vegetable oil in a 1:1 ratio; that is, dilute one drop of this synergistic blend in each milliliter of vegetable oil.

How Much Massage Oil to Use

For your massage, use only enough of the diluted blend to cover the hip and abdominal area. Of course, the amount you need will depend on your size. Use between 1 and 2 teaspoons of diluted oil per massage, making sure that enough of the blend is fully absorbed into the skin. If an oily residue remains on the skin after you complete the hip massage, use less oil next time.

How to Prepare the Massage Oil

Combine the essential oils by placing the correct amounts into a bottle and then rolling the bottle between your hands.

Then place the vegetable oil into the bottle, using a 1:1 ratio — that is, 1 milliliter of vegetable oil for each drop of essential oil. This ratio is approximately a 5 percent dilution. (To be precise, for an exact 5 percent dilution, add 1.5 milliliters of essential oil to 28.5 milliliters of vegetable oil.)

Put the lid on, turn the bottle upside down a few times, and then roll it vigorously between the palms of your hands. Label the bottle "Endometriosis Massage Oil" and add your name and the date. Each time, before you use the massage oil blend, roll the bottle between your hands for a few seconds. Spread the required amount of massage oil over your lower abdominal area, hips, and lower back.

The Massage Technique

1. Place your hands on your hips. Usually when people do this, the thumbs are at the back, and the four fingers are at the front of the body. Reverse this so your thumbs are at the front of your body.

2. Keeping your thumbs in this position, use all the fingers of both

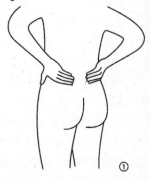

hands at the same time to massage in circular movements in the area between your hips and the crease of your buttocks.

3. Then massage around the sacrum area, the large bone at the base of the vertebrae, as if you were feeling the bone.

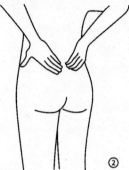

4. Applying pressure with your fingertips, massage in small circular movements along your hip, working toward the front of your body.

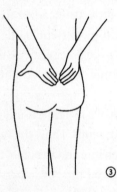

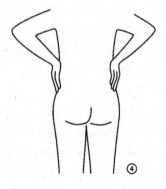

5. Put your hands on your hips again, in the more usual way — with your fingers to the front of your body. Use your thumbs this time to massage the lower back in small, circular movements, working toward the sacrum area and over the sacrum itself.

6. As you work your thumbs around the sacrum and down to the coccyx, you may find lumpy, nodulelike areas, which are often scar tissue: massage well over these. If you experience any

pain while massaging these areas, move over them gently and continue with the massage. You'll find that, after several days of massage and sitz bath treatments, the pain in these areas will go away. If it does not, speak to your doctor. (Remember, we are not treating back pain in general — that's another treatment entirely.)

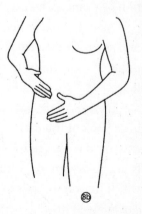

7. Place thumbs on either side of the vertebrae and pull the thumbs outward, toward the hips, applying pressure on the surface of the skin as you do so. Do this movement in straight lines, working from the waist to the crease in the buttocks, until you have covered the entire lower back area.

8. The last movement of the massage routine involves the lower abdomen. Use large, gentle circular movements with both of your hands. Start on your right side, by the pubic bone. Gradually work your way around

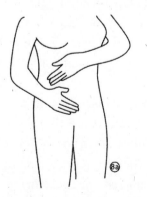

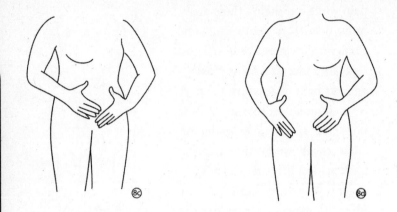

the abdomen as if you are following your colon, in a large clockwise circle, working across the diaphragm, and down the left side. By using both hands, this action will cover the whole of the abdomen. Repeat this movement several times. If you have any oil left on your hands, smooth it over the front and back of your thighs.

THE BATH AND SHOWER ROUTINE

Some women will not be able to purchase the equipment required to use the sitz bath routine. They can instead follow this bath and shower routine. However, this routine can also be used as an additional option by women who use the sitz bath and hip massage routines.

Water has the power to stimulate and relax us, and this stimulation and relaxation are part of the healing bath method. This is an 18-minute therapeutic routine that involves taking a 15-minute hot bath, followed by a 3-minute cold shower.

The idea of the hot bath is to relax as much as possible in it, reading a book or listening to music. The hot water dilates the capillaries and blood vessels, relaxing muscles and joints. Blood flow is increased, bringing oxygen to the internal organs. The heat causes perspiration, which is a way for the body to excrete toxins. For the hot bath, use the essential oils listed in the sidebar "Hot Bath Preparation."

HOT BATH PREPARATION

Blend together the following essential oils, then use 9 drops of the mixture for each hot bath.

	Thirty-day supply, for one bath per day:	Four-day supply, for one bath per day:
Geranium (*Pelargonium graveolens*)	4 milliliters	12 drops
Rose otto (*Rosa damascena*)	2 milliliters	6 drops
Cypress (*Cupressus sempervirens*)	1 milliliter	3 drops
Nutmeg (*Myristica fragrans*)	1 milliliter	3 drops
Clary sage (*Salvia sclarea*)	2 milliliters	6 drops
Helichrysum (*Helichrysum italicum*)	2 milliliters	6 drops

Make the temperature as hot as is comfortable for you, and add more hot water as needed to keep the temperature steady. You do not have to fill the bath up to the rim. It is just as effective if the water is at waist level. Hot water can affect blood pressure for a time, so if you feel at all dizzy get out of the bath.

After the hot bath, immediately take a cold shower. If you have a shower attachment, hold it against your abdomen and lower back. If you do not have a standing shower, use a tap shower attachment while sitting in the empty bath. Follow this with a hot shower over the same area as above.

PARTICULAR SYMPTOMS:
MASSAGE BLENDS AND OTHER METHODS

Bloating

If you experience abdominal bloating, especially premenstrually, substitute the Bloating Synergy Blend for Massage (see the sidebar) in place of the Endo Hip Massage Oil Blend, using the same massage technique (page 89) twice a day — morning and night. The essential oils in the following blend are helpful in reducing fluid retention.

THE NATURAL TREATMENT PROGRAM

BLOATING SYNERGY BLEND FOR MASSAGE

Cypress (*Cupressus sempervirens*)	5 drops
Caraway (*Carum carvi*)	2 drops
Rosemary (*Rosmarinus officinalis*)	3 drops
Juniper (*Juniperus communis*)	2 drops
Fennel (*Foeniculum vulgare* var. *dulce*)	2 drops

Blend the essential oils in a bottle in these proportions.

Dilute the synergy blend, using 1 milliliter of vegetable oil to each drop of synergy blend.

Bloating can be caused by several factors:

1. When the small capillaries are damaged by injury or pain, they release water into the body tissues. This process is called edema. The damage can be caused by a specific event, such as a blow to the body, or by inflammation, which is usually ongoing. The fluid leaking from damaged capillaries accumulates in the body's cavities, such as the peritoneal cavity, and the resulting swelling of the abdomen is often mistaken for digestive bloating. The release of histamine into the body during an allergic reaction can also cause fluid release and swelling.

2. Because digestive processes can affect hormone production, it is particularly important for women with endometriosis to maintain a healthy balance in their intestinal flora. The body plays host to millions of microorganisms, and no group should be allowed to dominate the others. The intestines can be kept in healthy balance by taking probiotics, which are a mixture of helpful bacteria such as *Bifidobacterium bifidum* and *Lactobacillus acidophilus*. If you suffer from much bloating, you might also consider taking

digestive enzymes. Use these supplements for a week or so to settle the digestive system before adding new elements to your diet.

3. Another possible cause of bloating, contradictory as it may seem, is dehydration. When the body is dehydrated it tries to hold on to any fluid it can, leading to water retention and bloating.

4. Although salt is vital for many biochemical processes of the body, most of us consume too much. As well as sprinkling it on our food, we consume it unwittingly not only in savory processed foods but also in unlikely sources such as chocolate and ice cream. It is also used as a thickener in many personal care products. According to nutritional advice, we should consume between one and three grams per day, but the average person consumes between three and seven grams. This can be a problem for those susceptible to hypertension, heart disease, and kidney problems and can also exacerbate fluid retention and bloating.

If you use processed salt with an anticaking agent added to it, change to a more natural option. Sea salt used to be ideal, until the oceans became polluted; now rock salt may be the better option. Potassium-rich foods can help to counteract any excess of salt (sodium) in the body.

Various supplements and herbs are recommended for bloating, including vitamin B6 (200 milligrams a day), borage oil, and magnesium. The herbal tinctures of chaste tree (*Vitex agnus castus*) and bearberry, also called uva ursi (*Arctostaphylos uva ursi*), help to some degree. A useful herbal tea to counteract bloating is peppermint.

Menstrual Uterine Cramps

During menstruation the uterus contracts to force the shedding endometrial lining through the cervix and into the vagina. These uterine contractions are experienced as "cramps." When you are experiencing these menstrual pains, use the Low-Abdominal-Pain Synergy Blend for Hip Massage on page 97 instead of the Endo Hip Massage Oil Blend on page 88, and use the massage technique described on pages 89–92.

Geranium essential oil can also be applied undiluted over the uterine area — use 2–3 drops, twice daily. As geranium has a pleasant roselike aroma, you can apply it during the day at work. Use this method when the monthly cramps are particularly severe.

A calcium-magnesium supplement may help with menstrual cramps, as may vitamin B6, vitamin E, and vitamin C with flavonoids. Vitamin D helps maintain calcium levels, which are lowest just before menstruation. Chamomile tea, which is calming, can also be helpful, as can ginger tea and raspberry leaf tea.

Low Abdominal Pain

Pain is one way the body can let us know something is wrong. It's a natural alert system, and it indicates that the problem has gone beyond the point at which the body can deal with it simply. Many women with endometriosis experience lower abdominal pain on nonmenstrual days. The pain is often described as a "twinge," while others say it is "knifelike." Every woman's experience is unique, but the pain is universal in that it is not related to the menstrual cycle — it comes on unexpectedly, and it hurts. Although the pain is often experienced on the lower left side of the abdomen, it could be felt anywhere in the abdominal area, depending on the woman's spread of endometrial implants, whether there is scar tissue, and the degree of inflammation. The Low-Abdominal-Pain Synergy Blend for Hip Massage (see the sidebar) can be used as a substitute for the daily Endo Hip Massage Oil Blend for a maximum of four days a month, if you find it more helpful. It has been formulated specifically to reduce painful symptoms. Return to the Endo Hip Massage Oil Blend as soon as the pain symptoms are alleviated.

LOW-ABDOMINAL-PAIN SYNERGY BLEND
FOR HIP MASSAGE

Basil (*Ocimum basilicum chemotype linalol*)	4 drops
Lavender (*Lavandula angustifolia*)	5 drops
Helichrysum (*Helichrysum italicum*)	9 drops
Nutmeg (*Myristica fragrans*)	2 drops
Cardamom (*Elettaria cardamomum*)	2 drops
Peppermint (*Mentha piperita*)	1 drop
Geranium (*Pelargonium graveolens*)	2 drops

Blend the essential oils in a bottle in these proportions.

Dilute the synergy blend, using 1 milliliter of vegetable oil to each 2 drops of the blend.

If the pain is making you feel particularly tense, add 2 drops of marjoram essential oil to the blend above, before diluting.

The sitz baths really help with lower abdominal pain. Some women are reluctant to take sitz baths when they are menstruating, but the baths are in fact very helpful in alleviating the pain of cramps, as well as nonmenstrual abdominal "twinges." If you really do not feel up to taking a sitz bath on certain days of the month, just place alternate hot and cold compresses on the abdominal area, in the form of an ice pack or a large bag of frozen peas alternating with a hot water bottle or warming pad. Hold each in place for 2 minutes. It is best to do this after having applied the Low-Abdominal-Pain Synergy Blend for Hip Massage.

Low Back Pain

If scar tissue has attached to the vertebra area, it can cause terrible pain felt most strongly just before and during menstruation. Heat applied to the affected area can ease the pain in some cases. Use a hot water bottle or a heating pad that can be heated in the microwave. Heating pads are also known as heat packs and may contain wheat, rice, and other natural products. It is not wise to put essential oils on these packs if you intend to put them in the microwave, because essential oils are flammable.

If heat does not relieve the pain, you could try a cold pack instead. This could simply be a pack of frozen peas that you keep specifically for this purpose. Make sure you wrap anything frozen in a piece of fabric before putting it against your bare skin.

Some essential oils are particularly effective for low back pain, such as those that have anti-inflammatory properties: for example, chamomile Roman (*Anthemis nobilis*), chamomile German (*Matricaria recutita*), lavender (*Lavandula angustifolia*), and peppermint (*Mentha piperita*), and muscle relaxants such as rosemary (*Rosmarinus officinalis*) and marjoram (*Origanum marjorana*).

A blend that may ease inflammatory pain is made up of equal parts of chamomile Roman, lavender, marjoram, and peppermint. Mix the essential oils together and apply 1–2 drops undiluted over the lower back, then cover the area with a small amount of vegetable oil.

Constipation

If endometrial implants and adhesions are attached to the organs of excretion, it can be extremely painful to urinate or defecate. The increasing buildup of fecal matter just puts more pressure on the internal organs and, possibly, the implants. Constipation is often the result of dehydration. If the stools are soft, it's much easier to pass them, and drinking lots of water during the day is the main way to help them become softer. It takes time for the body to absorb the water into fecal matter, produce softer stools, and start peristalsis (involuntary smooth muscle movement, such as of the intestines and colon).

Flaxseeds, oats, and dried fruits help many women. As you are more likely to get constipated around the time of your period, eat plenty of fruit and vegetables at this time. Flaxseeds can be sprinkled on breakfast cereals, on salads, and even on your lunchtime soup. The so-called green drinks or juices are also effective for intestinal balance when taken over a period of time. These include drinks that contain algae, spirulina, spinach, wheatgrass, and other dark green foods. Aloe vera juice is another option and may be helpful for those who experience stomach cramps or bowel disorders. Try to avoid any synthetic type of laxative, as these can create lazy bowel syndrome in those who use them over too long a period of time. Massaging over the intestinal tract in large circular clockwise movements often helps to move things along.

Diarrhea

Sudden bouts of diarrhea are most often the result of viral or bacterial infection, but chronic or ongoing diarrhea or loose bowels may indicate a food allergy or intolerance — to lactose (dairy) or wheat, for example. Parasitic infection, irritable bowel syndrome (IBS), and Crohn's disease are other possible causes. Shock, nervousness, and stress can also cause a problem. A B-vitamin deficiency can be responsible for chronic diarrhea, while too much vitamin C has the same effect. If the latter is the case, you've taken this vitamin beyond the point of "bowel tolerance."

A digestive enzyme deficiency can cause the food to pass undigested through the intestines, causing diarrhea. Probiotics help put friendly bacteria into the digestive system and are highly recommended in this case, along with a digestive enzyme supplement.

Because there are so many possibilities, it's important to find the cause of your diarrhea and treat it accordingly. Some women who have experienced loose bowels have been misdiagnosed as having irritable bowel syndrome and given medication for this when it was inappropriate. All possible causes must be discussed with your physician.

If you have chronic diarrhea and suffer continually from loose bowels, it's important to prevent dehydration by replacing the fluid, minerals, and electrolytes you are losing.

Digestive Disorders

There are many disorders that can give rise to excessive gas, bloating, bowel irritation, headache, abdominal pain, or feelings of sickness. Undetected food intolerances or a deficiency in digestive enzymes may be causing the gastric problems. An overgrowth of candida is another possible cause. Stress is one of the most common causes of digestive problems in men and women, and women with endometriosis have more than their fair share of that.

The first thing to do is to change to a balanced, organic diet. Eating smaller meals can help some people, as can avoiding drinks with your meals. Some nutritionists suggest that drinking liquids either before or after eating food is preferable to drinking them with your meal, because water and other drinks dilute the stomach's digestive juices, which cannot then do their job as effectively. Also, you might find it helpful to avoid spicy foods and acid-forming foods — such as carbohydrates and sugar. These are best eaten with vegetables, to give the proper pH balance.

Peppermint is excellent for flatulence, and it can be taken in many ways. A tincture of peppermint can be dropped in water, or you can take capsules that contain peppermint oil. There is also peppermint tea; other tea options include ginger root tea, fennel tea, and cardamom tea.

Essential oils are among the best things for digestive problems, and they are found in many natural digestive supplements derived from plants. Any of the essential oils listed in the Digestion-Aid Massage Blend (see the sidebar) will help when used on their own in a massage oil. Alternatively, try massaging the blend over the upper abdomen and stomach area.

DIGESTION-AID MASSAGE BLEND

Dill (*Anethum graveolens*)	1 drop
Cardamom (*Elettaria cardamomum*)	2 drops
Coriander (*Coriandrum sativum*)	2 drops

Dilute in 1 teaspoon of vegetable oil.

Fatigue

One of the problems with having a condition such as endometriosis is that everything is blamed on it. Fatigue is a case in point. Of course women with endometriosis are going to feel fatigued. Coping with any sort of pain is exhausting and, if you have endometriosis, just knowing that every month it will relentlessly return can wear you down. The fatigue is both physical and emotional. Along with the effort of dealing with the physical pain, there is the stress of learning to live with endometriosis. But although there are many reasons why endometriosis can make you feel exhausted, this doesn't mean the tiredness you feel is inevitably one of its results. Fatigue may be caused by thyroid problems, hormonal problems, diabetes, or one of many other conditions that you should be evaluated for — so they can either be treated or ruled out. This is why it's always important to mention fatigue to your physician, recognizing it as a specific symptom, not just an inevitability of your life as an endometriosis sufferer.

A common cause of fatigue is a bad diet, one full of "dead" food such as cakes, instead of "live" food, such as fruits, nuts, seeds, and raw vegetables. Try changing to a healthier diet and drinking plenty of still mineral water, and see if this gives you an unexpected surge of energy. If you already have a predominantly "live" diet, and still feel fatigued, speak to your physician about potential causes.

THE NATURAL TREATMENT PROGRAM

Headaches and Migraines

Headaches are very, very seldom a symptom of something serious like a brain tumor. They are much more likely to occur as a result of dehydration, hunger, irregular meals, bad posture, overexcitement, or a change in the weather. If they occur on a regular basis, you should consult your physician to see if you have high or low blood pressure.

Migraines are extremely serious headaches that can be completely debilitating. They can be brought on by certain foods — cheese, chocolate, citrus fruits, and red wine being the main culprits. Some people are particularly sensitive to food additives, and all migraine sufferers should keep a food diary to try and identify if there are any food or food additive triggers.

There are two types of migraine: the classic, which is characterized by visual disturbances and a throbbing headache in one particular area of the head, nausea, and vomiting. With this type, objects often appear to have an aura — sparkling lights — around them. This can give rise to a temporary reduction of vision, which can last from several minutes to over an hour. With classic migraine, the eyes become so sensitive to light that relief can be found only by resting in a darkened room.

The common migraine, also called gastric migraine, affects mainly one side of the head, or the front or the back of the head. There is throbbing pain, sometimes accompanied by nausea and vomiting. This type starts slowly and gradually develops. It can lead to temporary numbness of one side of the face, head, and neck.

Common triggers of migraine are stress, allergies, food intolerances, and hormonal changes. In women with endometriosis who experience migraine, it usually happens just before menstruation or when ovulating.

The cooling essential oils are recommended for both headaches and migraines. The Headache- and Migraine-Cooling Gel (see the sidebar) blend can be prepared in advance and kept in the refrigerator, ready for when needed. Only use a small amount of the gel, applied on both temples and the back of the neck along the hairline, making sure you avoid the eye area.

HEADACHE- AND MIGRAINE-COOLING GEL

Rosemary (*Rosmarinus officinalis*)	5 drops
Peppermint (*Mentha piperita*)	3 drops
Lavender (*Lavandula angustifolia*)	2 drops
Chamomile Roman (*Anthemis nobilis*)	2 drops
Eucalyptus (*Eucalyptus radiata*)	4 drops

Mix well with 10 grams (2 teaspoons) of aloe vera gel.

Aspirin was originally derived from the bark of a willow tree, and even today women gain enormous relief from white willow, which is sold in capsules in health stores. The herb feverfew is helpful for both headaches and migraines. It can be obtained in either capsule or tincture form. If you find that feverfew gives you relief, you might consider growing it in the garden, where you can pick the leaves, when required, to make a tea, or simply add the leaves to salads. For women with gastric migraine and nausea, ginger supplements can be very useful, as can ginger and peppermint teas.

Hemorrhoids

When the veins in the lining of the anus swell, the swellings are known as hemorrhoids. They often come from straining to pass fecal matter, which is in turn caused by constipation or by having hard stools. Signs of hemorrhoids are rectal bleeding, pain on passing feces, and sometimes discharge from the anus and itching. If you have any of these symptoms, you must visit your physician and get an accurate diagnosis, because these symptoms can indicate much more serious conditions.

Drink plenty of water to keep the body hydrated and the stools soft. Rubbing a combination of diluted cypress and geranium essential oils around the anal area often alleviates the discomfort. Dilute 5 drops of each essential oil in 10 milliliters ($^1/_3$ fluid ounce) of vegetable oil.

Insomnia

Insomnia is common among women with endometriosis, perhaps because their pain keeps them awake, or perhaps because they lie and worry about finding a solution to their condition. Or it may be that the endometriosis affects other aspects of their lives, and they worry about that. Whatever the cause, there is perhaps nothing as desolate as lying in the dark, feeling heavy as lead, exhausted, desperate to sleep but unable to do so. It's a frustrating waste of time and annoying because you know your body needs to sleep to be able to heal.

Insomnia makes it difficult to get through the days. You are likely to feel fatigued and irritable. It is no consolation to know that one in three people suffer from it at some time in their lives. All you can think is, "Will I be able to sleep tonight?"

Taking sleeping pills is not a great option for women with endometriosis, because they may well be taking other medication. It would be better to look for natural alternatives and lifestyle strategies that may break the insomnia habit. Each woman will have to find her own solution to the problem, because we are all unique, and what works for some women will not work for all. Try the following options until you find what works for you.

- Take warm baths at night. Adding 4–6 drops of lavender essential oil can have a calming, sleep-inducing effect on some women. Another essential oil with calming and soothing effects is neroli (*Citrus aurantium*). Use 1–2 drops in a bath.
- Read in bed. Use light reading material — no scary novels or textbooks.
- Play relaxing music on a CD player; set the device to turn off after a period of time.

- Drink calming teas before bedtime: chamomile, linden blossom, lime blossom, orange blossom, lemon balm (melissa), or valerian.
- Put 2 drops of lavender, or 1 drop of neroli, on your pillow — on the side, or under the corner, away from your eyes.
- Put a mug of steaming hot water near your bed, and add the following essential oils:

Valerian	1 drop
Lavender	2 drops
Chamomile	3 drops

- Just before bed, take tincture of passiflora, valerian root, or hops — all of which have a calming effect.
- Avoid stimulants after 6 p.m. — such as alcohol, tea, coffee, sodas with caffeine, and sugar.
- Change your routine after work. This would be a good time to do the gentle exercise routines required by the self-help treatment program.

CALMING ESSENTIAL OILS

For a calming effect, try one of the following essential oils in an oil burner, room fragrancer, or essential oil diffuser:

- Valerian (*Valeriana officinalis*)
- Neroli (*Citrus aurantium*)
- Lavender (*Lavandula angustifolia*)
- Chamomile Roman (*Anthemis nobilis*)
- Hops (*Humulus lupulus*)
- Melissa (*Melissa officinalis*)
- Marjoram (*Origanum marjorana*)
- Clary sage (*Salvia sclarea*)
- Yarrow (*Achillea millefolium*)
- Vetiver (*Vetiveria zizanoides*)

Tension

Everyone gets tense at times, but women with endometriosis get tense more often than most, simply because they have so much to deal with physically and emotionally. As we know, endometriosis can affect all aspects of a woman's life. Sometimes it's just too much, and it may seem that the only way out is to go to bed, pull the covers over your head, and hide from the world. Unfortunately you can't always do this, and you just have to get on with life. Tension can build gradually, and you may find yourself unable to relax, irritable, hostile, angry, unable to make decisions, and generally barely able to cope. This is life on the edge, and it's a very uncomfortable place to be.

TENSION-RELIEVING BLEND

Neroli (*Citrus aurantium*)	6 drops
Orange (*Citrus sinensis*)	3 drops
Bergamot (*Citrus aurantium bergamia*)	1 drop

Blend together in these proportions and use 4 drops in a bath. Or dilute this amount in 10 milliliters ($\frac{1}{3}$ fluid ounce) of vegetable oil and use up to 5 milliliters of the mixture on the body, in the morning or at night.

This blend will relieve tension, whether you are on the self-help program or not. If you can't obtain these particular essential oils, you could use any of the following tension-relieving essential oils diluted on their own — 1 drop of essential oil diluted in 1 milliliter of vegetable oil:

Neroli (*Citrus aurantium*)
Bergamot (*Citrus aurantium bergamia*)
Geranium (*Pelargonium graveolens*)
Rose otto (*Rosa damascena*)
Grapefruit (*Citrus paradisi*)

Endometriosis often brings with it a sense of sheer frustration, a feeling that this problem will never be resolved, that life will never change for the better. It is this which gives rise to so much tension, and if endometriosis goes on for a very long time, these feelings of tension can become a habit. Unfortunately, tension exacerbates the symptoms of endometriosis, and having everyone tell you to "relax" can make matters worse.

Certain essential oils are well known for being among the most effective ways of dealing with tension. Their effect can be dramatic — in the nicest, most gentle way. The Tension-Relieving Blend (see the sidebar) has a particularly pleasant aroma, and as it reduces feelings of tension, it will help put things in perspective.

HERBS

Many women have found that certain herbs alleviate the symptoms of endometriosis. Choose herbs that have an action best suited to your own symptoms or problem areas. Peppermint, for example, is particularly good for women with digestive problems, including ir-ritable bowel syndrome. Milk thistle is excellent as part of a detoxi-fication program because it strengthens the liver. Agnus castus has traditionally been used to regulate hormones and the menstrual cycle. This, in turn, can reduce symptoms such as mood swings and anxiety. It's not wise to take more than three herbal remedies at any given time, however.

Agnus Castus (Chaste Berry) (Vitex agnus castus)

The chaste tree is actually a shrub producing violet-colored flowers, and its berries are the source of the agnus castus. They are very dark red in color and resemble peppercorns. Once found only around the Mediterranean, the chaste tree is now cultivated in various subtrop-ical areas of the world. It is a pretty plant that can be grown in the gar-den and is easily propagated.

This herb is widely used in Europe for premenstrual syndrome.

According to some reports, the chaste berry works by stimulating the pituitary gland, which then produces a greater amount of luteinizing hormone (LH), which prompts the ovaries to produce progesterone. While the chaste berry is not a phytoestrogen itself, it causes hormonal effects, appearing to encourage a more normal balance of estrogen and progesterone.

For women trying to become pregnant, and who have been diagnosed with luteal phase defect, chaste berry may be very helpful. In addition to balancing estrogen and progesterone, it lowers prolactin, a hormone produced by the pituitary gland. Do check with your physician, however, before using it during the menstrual cycle, as opinions differ on whether this is healthful. Cease taking the herb if you become pregnant.

Dosages

Chaste berry is available as a dried herb, powdered extract, tea, tablet or capsule, liquid extract, or tincture. The active ingredient is agnuside.

Daily recommended dosages:
- Powdered extract: 200–400 milligrams (agnuside should be included to .5 percent).
- Tincture: 20 drops 3 times a day in $\frac{1}{4}$ cup of water, before meals.
- Liquid extract: 1 teaspoon 3 times a day.

Can be taken alongside vitamin B6 if PMS symptoms are very bad.

Cease taking after 6 months if you are treating PMS, and 1 year if you are treating fertility problems.

Contraindications

Not to be taken at the same time as any hormonal drugs, including contraceptives.

Not to be taken at the same time as drugs that include bromocriptine, which inhibits secretion of the hormone prolactin, or those that affect dopamine secretion. These include antipsychotics and drugs for Parkinson's disease.

Not to be taken if you have a history of miscarriage.

Not to be taken if you are pregnant.

Not to be taken while you are breastfeeding, as it lowers milk production through its effect on the hormone prolactin.

Not to be taken if you are undergoing in vitro fertilization treatments, as it lowers the follicle-stimulating hormone (FSH).

Cease taking chaste berry if it increases menstrual flow (unless this is desired), or if there is any discomfort in the stomach, or if you develop itchy skin.

Peppermint (Mentha piperita)

The peppermint plant, with its prolific leaf growth and tiny purple flowers arranged in cone-shaped clumps, will take over any flowerbed, given half a chance. It's widely used around the world as peppermint tea. The leaves are harvested just before the flowers bloom. Cultivation in the United States began around 1850.

Peppermint is probably best known as a digestive aid: it is a carminative, which relieves flatulence and, with it, abdominal pain and bloating; and it is an antispasmodic, which reduces muscle spasm. Peppermint is also said to encourage the secretion and flow of bile, which removes waste from the liver, allowing it to be processed and eliminated by the body.

Dosages

Take as directed on the packaging. Daily recommended dosages:
- Tincture: 15 drops 3 times a day in $1/4$ cup of water, before meals.
- Tea: as often as you want.

Contraindications

Not to be used by those with hiatal hernia, as it may make acid reflux worse.

Milk Thistle (Silybum marianum)

This decorative plant, native to Southeast Asia, southern Europe, and North Africa, produces a distinctive, large purple thistle. The Bedouins of the Sahara Desert in North Africa find a use for the young shoots, but it is the seeds that are generally used medicinally. They encourage the secretion and flow of bile and have been shown in scientific tests to have a positive effect on the liver. When there is inefficient bile secretion, the liver becomes sluggish and gallstones form more easily.

This is the herb of choice for protecting the liver against damage and encouraging the production of new cells. It enhances the liver's ability to work efficiently and aids in detoxification. It contains the flavone silymarin — which is an excellent antioxidant, as well as silydianin and silychristin. If you are, or have been, a heavy alcohol drinker or on drugs or medications, milk thistle will help clear the liver of toxins. As an antioxidant, milk thistle is said to be ten times more effective than vitamin E.

While carrying out a detoxification plan, eat organic produce as far as you can. Avoid dairy products, wheat, and meat — to avoid the hormones and growth enhancers animals are fed with. Cut out all meats including animals reared organically. Fish can be eaten, but no more than three times a week, along with plenty of organic fruits and vegetables, including cabbage. Avoid alcohol, coffee, and tea, including green tea. Drink plenty of bottled water, which will help you avoid constipation. Try not to hold your urine in: go to the bathroom as often as required. Vitamin C helps at this time. You may feel a little nauseated when first starting the detoxification program — be prepared for this, and don't let it put you off continuing.

Dosages

Milk thistle can be purchased in tincture or tablet form. Take according to the directions on the packaging. Daily recommended dosages:

- Tincture: 10 drops 2 times a day, working up to 10 drops 3 times a day, in $^1/_4$ cup of water, before meals.
- Tablets: as indicated on the packaging.

Drink lots of water at the same time to help the elimination system along.

Contraindications
None known.

NUTRITIONAL SUPPLEMENTS

There are so many nutritional supplements available these days that it can be difficult to decide what to take, if anything. Professional guidance is always the best option; however, the following supplements will help prepare the body to heal itself and can be taken by women with endometriosis.

A good multivitamin would probably benefit anyone, and individual women may benefit from additional vitamins B6 and E. Some women will find a combined magnesium-calcium supplement useful. A deficiency in connective tissue can be counteracted by selenium, while zinc can help if your immunity is low and you're experiencing a lot of coughs and colds. If you are trying to get pregnant, combine the zinc with vitamin E. Bear in mind that zinc is absorbed only if taken at night. If you are feeling stressed, not sleeping well, or on a lot of medication, B complex is helpful. Vitamin C always helps the healing process.

Please refer to chapter 10 for detailed information on these and other nutritional supplements.

REDUCING STRESS

Evaluate your current stress levels by completing the chart on the next page.

- Please mark the degree of stress you experience in various areas of your life, on a scale of 0 to 5, with 5 being very high.

- If you mark any area 3 or higher, write a brief reason why in the box to the right.
- Use the spare rows to insert other areas of stress particular to your life.

STRESS LEVELS IN YOUR LIFE							
	0	1	2		3	4	5	Reason
Work							
Travel							
Partner							
Children							
Other Family — past							
Other Family — present							
Ill Health							
Home Environment							
Education/Study							
Friends							

If there are people in your life who cause you stress, try to avoid them. Don't invite them over, and don't return their phone calls unless you have to. You may choose not to tell these people that you are taking up this self-help program.

It's generally advisable to cut down on the number of people you see to allow yourself to focus on what you are experiencing and achieving. Take this time for yourself, and concentrate on your needs instead of everyone else's.

A great way to relax is to go out more. Go out once a week with a friend for a quiet dinner or for a quiet walk. Spend some time thinking about the list above. What can you do to change your situation? Carry out just one small thing a day, and work toward reducing the stressful areas of your life.

SEXUALITY

If there are endometrial implants on the uterosacral ligaments — which attach to each side of the uterus — intercourse can be extremely painful. As the penis pushes into the vagina, pressure is exerted on the cervix, uterus, and uterosacral ligaments. With each push these ligaments are strained, and any endometrial implants on or near them are stressed. Inflammation may follow.

Endometrial implants can be anywhere in the abdominal cavity, and only the woman herself knows whether they hurt during sex and what kind of sex is painful. For this reason, you should have the last word as to what sexual activity is okay.

In this self-help treatment program, you do quite a bit of preparatory work before undertaking the more proactive phase, which is when you use the essential oils (or homeopathy, herbs, or acupuncture, and so on). During this preparatory time, carry on with your usual sexual activity, but when you begin the essential-oil strand of the program — if you are sexually active — refrain from intercourse for one full menstrual cycle. Other, less vigorous sexual activity can be enjoyed at this time.

EVALUATING PERSONAL CARE PRODUCTS

The next step in the program is to look at the chemicals you apply on or near your body on a daily basis. This includes products connected with menstruation, as well as cosmetics, skin creams, body lotions, perfumes, sunscreens, and hair products.

Methods of blood analysis are now so sophisticated that we know our bodies are like sponges soaking up chemicals from the personal care products we use every day, as well as from the food we eat and the air we breathe, both inside and outside the home. The question is not "Do we absorb chemicals?" but "How exactly did this cocktail of chemicals get inside me?" For example, parabens have been found in breast cancer tumors, according to researchers at Reading University in the United Kingdom (Darbre 2004), but the question is, "Did they get there through the use of deodorants and other personal care products, by means of the foods we have eaten, or by some other route?"

Parabens are used as preservatives in a wide range of personal care products. Research has shown that they create an estrogenic effect on the uteruses of rats, but not when the parabens are given by mouth, only when they are applied on the skin or administered under the skin. The significance of this is that an overload of estrogens, whether naturally occurring in the body or synthetically created, has been hypothesized as the cause of endometriosis. Whether or not this is the case, parabens also have been shown to disrupt the function of cells by inhibiting the secretion of lysosomal enzymes, and to cause dysfunction in mitochondria, the powerhouses found in every cell.

Research in Denmark found parabens in 99 percent of leave-on personal care products and 77 percent of rinse-off ones. Another, earlier study showed parabens to be components of 13,200 products. Parabens are in widespread use in face moisturizers and body lotions, for example. The names to look for in the ingredient lists of personal care products are: methyl paraben, propyl paraben, benzyl paraben, ethyl paraben, and isobutyl paraben.

A new vocabulary is emerging. Your "body burden" describes the number and amount of chemicals you have absorbed. Some chemicals are more "bioaccumulative" than others — they are more likely to accumulate in us. Chemicals can "biomagnify" through the food chain.

Several studies have shown that human beings in the industrialized world have absorbed around three hundred different chemicals. As most are incorporated into a variety of products, it's difficult to establish how an individual chemical becomes absorbed by a particular body. The general consensus, however, is that it's better for an individual to have a "body burden" as small as possible. Clearly, the fewer chemicals used in the production of your food, used to clean your home, contained in the structure of your home, applied to your garden, emanating from your furniture upholstery, or used directly on your body, the better. When it comes to the subject of synthetic chemicals, less is definitely best. For a woman with endometriosis, the chemicals of particular concern are those that disrupt hormones or interfere with functioning of the liver, thyroid gland, and immune system.

Phthalates (phthalate esters) are produced in many chemical forms and are known to be toxic to the reproductive system. Previously, they were added to cosmetics and perfumes as solvents or thinners — until they were implicated in the development of cancer and banned. At least, this was the case in countries where there is regulation in this field. Products from less-developed countries may still contain phthalates, and, of course, older women used products containing phthalates for years before the potential dangers to health were realized.

With synthetic chemicals, legislation usually works around the idea that a substance is safe unless challenged and then proven unsafe. According to this principle, a chemical additive is "innocent until proven guilty." In a strategy for a future chemicals policy published by the European Commission in February 2001, the commission notes that Europe is not alone in having an uncontrolled chemical industry: "Government agencies in Canada and the United States have recently launched initiatives to acquire testing data for large numbers of chemical substances currently on their markets in high volumes on which little is known about the risks. In fact, not one country has yet been successful in overcoming the huge gap in knowledge of substances." The report also states, "The lack of knowledge about the impact of many chemicals on human health and the environment is a cause for concern."

Menstrual Care Products

Most tampons and sanitary napkins are bright white because they've been bleached with chlorine. Any chemical residue on them may put women at risk, since these products are placed against the delicate genital mucous membrane and, in the case of tampons, inside the vagina, with its highly absorbent membrane lining. The issue of bleached sanitary products has been of long-standing concern to environmental groups, who point out that these products have residues of chlorine, dioxins, and the pesticides used in the agricultural production of cotton.

The manufacturing process of personal care products also creates dioxins, which are released into the environment. Dioxins have been implicated in the development of endometriosis in baboons. Fortunately, tampons and sanitary napkins made of organic, unbleached materials are available in health shops and supermarkets — and women with endometriosis should consider using them.

Hair Products

Regular use of permanent hair dyes that include arylamines has been linked to an increased risk of developing cancer. Natural henna is an alternative colorant for dark-haired women, and fresh lemon juice in the final rinse water gives a shine to blond hair. Hairsprays may contain damaging chemical particles, and these are inhaled during application. Many hair wax products, including conditioners for Afro-Caribbean hair, contain mineral oil (liquid paraffin — paraffinum liquidum). Natural alternatives to this petroleum product are available that work well and cause no harm to the hair or environment.

Cosmetics

It's often said that most of the lipstick we apply eventually ends up in our mouths and digestive systems. If that's the case, we are actually consuming parabens, propylene glycol, and lanolin, among other components. Arsenic was previously a common component of eye shadow, and although the amount used may have been very small, arsenic interferes with hormones — and the skin on the eyelid is very thin and therefore absorbent. Face powder may contain titanium dioxide, which has been deemed a potential carcinogen. Foundation, moisturizers, and mascara often contain parabens, which mimic estrogens. Our exposure to these and other chemicals is chronic: on a daily basis, all day every day. Although, taken individually, these components constitute a very small quantity, they come in a cocktail of other chemical components and are usually used in conjunction with several other products. A woman with endometriosis might be well advised to assess what she is putting on her face, and to look for alternatives produced by the growing number of manufacturers who attempt to replace the harmful chemical components.

Nail Products

Nails are porous and may absorb compounds included in varnish, removers, and strengtheners. Three chemicals that have been shown to have an effect on health when used in large quantities are toluene, acetone, and formaldehyde. Women working in the field of nail care, and especially those applying acrylic and other false nails, need additionally to be aware of the health dangers associated with methyl methacrylate (MMA), benzoyl peroxide, and hydroquinone.

Antiperspirants and Deodorants

The preservatives used in deodorants and antiperspirants sometimes contain parabens, which, as noted earlier, have been found inside breast cancer tumors. Because of the proximity of the underarm to the tumor, it has been speculated that deodorants and antiperspirants are to blame. But parabens are used in so many products that it's actually impossible to know which personal care product or even food was the source of these particular parabens.

However, we might ask, "Do we really need deodorants or antiperspirants?" We know that sweating is a natural body function because it is a form of excretion and helps control body temperature. At the same time we don't want to smell! Fortunately, natural deodorants are available, and washing the underarms twice a day is always an option.

Sunscreens

The chemicals in sunscreens, released into the environment as people swim in the sea, can damage offshore banks of coral. This tells us that these are powerful products — and they have to be to prevent the sun's ultraviolet rays from damaging the skin.

Swiss researchers have found that five chemicals commonly used in sunscreens mimic estrogen, and at least one has shown up in breast milk — indicating that it's accumulating in the body. The skin's outer layer is our natural barrier against ultraviolet rays, but many skin products peel away this layer to reveal a smoother, more youthful look. This leaves us more vulnerable to ultraviolet rays, which is one reason manufacturers often incorporate sunscreens into these skin products.

Some moisturizers that incorporate sun protection ingredients are marketed for both day and night use. Given that we don't need sun protection at night, it might be wise to avoid this unnecessary nighttime exposure to extra chemicals.

The Way Forward

If you go on a healing program to detoxify yourself, it makes sense to evaluate what personal care products you are using at the moment. This is not an easy task, unless you are a professional chemist and know which of the components with long ingredient names are natural and which are synthetic, and which of the synthetic chemicals might be hormone disruptors or might affect the healthy working of your immune system, thyroid gland, or liver. There is a long learning curve with this subject, and all any of us can do is try to move in the right direction and become more aware of what we are putting on our faces and bodies. Environmental pressure groups are often a good source of information.

EVALUATING SOCIAL HABITS

We all know that certain habits are bad for us, such as smoking, drinking alcohol, and eating too much fat and sugar, especially in the form of chocolate and other candy. Yet we continue to indulge in these habits. They are hard to give up, despite endless advice that we should do so. Since you already know that cigarettes are full of harmful chemicals, alcohol hurts the liver, and an overabundance of sugar is detrimental and forces your body to work harder, you don't need to be told again.

A very good catchphrase states that "this is the first day of the rest of your life." You can adopt this the day you decide to stop your own bad social habit. It really is true that the day a person stops smoking is a landmark day. Deciding to order a glass of orange juice instead of a glass of wine is a big step. Saying no to a chocolate bar at the supermarket checkout stand is a brave move. Have a reward system in place: put the money you would have spent on your bad social habit in a jar, save it up, and buy yourself a treat.

EVALUATING HOUSEHOLD AND GARDEN PRODUCTS

Polar bears on the Arctic ice pack are contaminated with the same perfluorinated compounds that are used in food packaging, textiles, and the coating on nonstick pans. According to a 2004 World Wildlife Fund (WWF) report, these cancer-causing chemicals are also found in dolphins, seals, and whales.

The WWF is extremely concerned about the effect that the more than thirty thousand chemicals in general use are having on animals — and we should be worried about the effect they are having on us too. Investigation into chemical exposure within the home is a relatively new science, and it is revealing a host of potential health hazards. According to some research, there is ten times more pollution inside the average home than outside it. This pollution comes from the chemicals used in carpets, furniture, carpentry glues, household cleaning chemicals, and many other sources. The presence of these chemicals can be measured in human urine and in air and dust samples.

According to a 2003 report, more than sixty hormone-disrupting chemicals and twenty-seven pesticides were found in samples taken from 120 homes in the Cape Cod area of Massachusetts, as well as in the urine of the study's participants (Rudel et al. 2003). In their study, the authors of the report had targeted various chemicals for analysis, including phthalates, parabens, alkylphenols, polybrominated biphenyl ethers, polyaromatic hydrocarbons, polychlorinated biphenyls (PCBs), bisphenol A, and other estrogenic phenols.

A similar 2003 study by the Greenpeace Research Laboratories found an abundance of chemicals in the dust of homes across Britain (Santillo et al. 2003). The report states, "Chemicals that may present a long-term hazard to human health are present in significant amounts in virtually every one of over 100 homes we visited. Here then is a clue as to why levels are increasing, exponentially in some cases, in human breast milk, blood and other body tissues."

Also in 2003, the reproductive sciences unit of the United Kingdom's Medical Research Council published the results of a two-year experiment in which rats were exposed to phthalates. Researchers found that phthalates disrupt the hormone testosterone, doubling the rate of defects and reducing sperm counts (Sharpe and Irvine 2004).

All the evidence points in the same direction: we are in danger of chemical overload and must reduce our intake by all possible means. We will still have a body burden of chemicals, because they cannot all be avoided, but at least it will be smaller. If you suspect you have a chemical overload, perhaps due to your working environment, specific tests are available for a variety of pesticides, organophosphates, solvents, plastics, plasticizers, silicones, food additives, metals, halogens including fluoride, and environmental chemicals such as PCBs, exhaust fumes, and formaldehyde.

Household Insect Pests

There is a world of household insects, ranging from the scary but harmless spider to the cockroach that comes out at night. Not all insects can be dealt with by the "jar and postcard" method — in which you catch the insect in a small container, put a postcard over the opening, and release the insect outside unharmed. Unfortunately, insect infestations do occur. Increasingly there are mechanical products available that catch insects for humane release. If you cannot find an appropriate product, then manual means of control are generally preferable to chemical means. In simple terms, "catch, don't spray."

Insects have a natural habitat — and it is not your home. In nature, they live outside. What we must do is deter them from coming into the home in the first place, and a number of products oriented toward deterrence have come onto the market. Chemical sprays in the home linger. The droplets fall on carpets, on which babies might crawl. While spraying, you might inhale the chemicals. And analysis of household dust shows that insecticides are still around us long after the insects have gone.

Doormats

The simple doormat can greatly reduce the amount of lead brought into the house from the outside urban environment. What would be better still is to also remove your shoes before entering your home. Find a cupboard to put by the door so shoes can be put out of sight.

Furniture

One group of chemicals highlighted by both the WWF and Greenpeace as being of particular environmental and health concern includes the brominated flame retardants used in electronic goods and furniture. These are known to mimic thyroid hormones, which is unhelpful to women with endometriosis. We know these chemicals do not stay locked in plastics or furniture, because they show up in house dust. The difficulty is that we all have electronic goods and furniture, and it's difficult to see how we can avoid inhaling or touching these chemicals. Perhaps our only hope in this regard is to impress upon our legislators the need to change regulations that govern the manufacture of goods incorporating brominated flame retardants.

Flooring

Carpets are often treated with chemicals designed to kill mold or dust mites. Vinyl (PVC) flooring is made soft and pliable by the use of phthalates. Of these, di-2-ethyl hexyl phthalate (DEHP) is the most widely used, and it's a known reproductive toxin. Its toxicity to the male reproductive system has been known for over fifty years. It also affects liver function, immune function, and hormone metabolism — functions especially important to women with endometriosis. Wooden floors seem the safest option, but the varnish applied on them should be chosen carefully.

Cleaning Products

A group of chemicals widely used in industrial detergents, in pesticides, and in textile and leather finishing, among other applications, are the alkylphenols and their derivatives. Of these, Greenpeace says, "The most widely recognised hazard associated with [them] is undoubtedly their oestrogenic activity, i.e., their ability to mimic natural oestrogen hormones. This can lead to altered sexual development in some organisms, most notably the feminisation of fish" (Santillo et al. 2003). These chemicals also appear to damage the DNA in human lymphocytes.

There are, fortunately, many natural alternatives to chemical cleaning products. Vinegar can be used to clean windows and descale taps. Bicarbonate of soda (sodium hydrogen carbonate) is an effective surface cleaner and can be used straight or diluted with water. Many tips on natural cleaning alternatives, using lemon juice, essential oils, and olive oil, for example, can be found in books or on the Internet. Adopting alternative cleaning products to any extent is a step in the right direction, both for our health and for the environment.

Candles

Most candles, including the so-called aromatherapy candles, are made from petrochemical waxes such as paraffin and incorporate synthetic chemicals and perfumes. When the candle is lit, toxic pollutants such as soot and volatile organic compounds are released into the air. If the room is not well ventilated, the compounds are inhaled. Look for beeswax, soya wax, and other natural candles.

Food Storage

Xenoestrogens (chemicals that mimic the hormone estrogen) are often contained in the plastics formed into plastic bottles and food containers, and they leach into food. Plastic food wrapping may also be problematic. Whenever possible, buy drinks in glass bottles and, if food is purchased already packaged in plastic wrapping of any kind, remove it as soon as possible when you get home. This is especially the case for fatty foods such as cheese and meat.

The Garden

Most of us have grown up in a world where applying chemicals in the garden is normal. Garden centers offer row upon row of chemical concoctions designed to annihilate any small creature that moves on the flowers, bushes, or lawn. Much of this carnage can be avoided by careful "companion planting" — placing side-by-side the plants that naturally protect each other, either by deterring particular insects by changing the chemical structure of the soil, by allowing more light or shade, or by creating a particular aromatic environment. This is a gentle science in its own right, on which much has been written.

Most often, stressed plants are the ones susceptible to insect attack. Plants resist insect invasion — and disease — when they're well fed and properly watered, and when they receive the correct amount of sunlight for their species. Creating and maintaining healthy soil takes a little bit of work, but it's not hard to do and it leads to healthy plants.

CHAPTER EIGHT

Complementary Therapies for Endometriosis

A physician practices allopathic medicine, also known as ortho-dox medicine. This usually involves treating the patient with pharmaceutical drugs or surgery. One criticism of this system is that it treats the symptoms rather than the cause of the problem. For example, if you go to a doctor with psoriasis, a skin condition that often flares up during periods of stress, he or she may prescribe a cream to be applied on the skin. Complementary systems of medicine tend to be more broad-based, and a practitioner will look at the patient's personality, emotional state, dietary habits, and whole lifestyle, as well as physical symptoms, before deciding which approach to take in the treatment.

About twenty years ago, people used the term *alternative medicine* to describe any system of healing different from that offered by physicians. Pretty soon it became clear that the word *alternative* wasn't appropriate, because it implied there was an "either-or" choice — you went either to a doctor, or to an alternative practitioner. In fact, many people went to both. These "extra" systems of healthcare complemented orthodox medicine in that they could work well together. The term *complementary* came to be seen as more appropriate than *alternative*, although both words actually describe the same thing.

As the practice of complementary medicine gets wider, the vocabulary has expanded. The term *holistic medicine* simply means that the patient is seen as a whole person — body, mind, and spirit — and everything works together as an integrated unit. The term *integrative medicine* is used when orthodox and complementary medicines are practiced in the same clinic or hospital. A patient might be treated with modern medicine or surgery, as well as with one or more of the complementary therapies, depending on what is most appropriate. Often several systems are integrated into treatment.

Certain branches of complementary healing are complete systems of medicine in themselves and have their own methods of diagnosis and treatment: homeopathy and Ayurvedic medicine fall into this group. Then there are therapies that use orthodox diagnosis and treat the condition based on that information — such is the case with aromatherapy. A few of the complementary systems are not treatments as such but diagnostic tools — iridology, for example, in which the iris of the eye is examined. Another group of practices could really be called self-help systems, such as breathing techniques, nutritional therapy, Alexander technique, and yoga. These can all be taught to you, but essentially they are knowledge that is under your own control and that you put into practice in your own time.

Each system of complementary therapy has its strengths and advantages and areas where it really cannot help a particular symptom or medical condition. Success in using complementary therapies in general depends a great deal on choosing a system that is appropriate to the particular medical problem for which you are seeking help. In this section we highlight complementary therapies that some women have found helpful in the treatment of endometriosis. They are herbalism, Chinese herbs, Ayurveda, bodywork techniques including massage, acupuncture, hydrotherapy, homeopathy, biochemic cell salts, flower remedies, and naturopathy.

Most people turn to complementary medicine as a last resort, having tried everything the doctor has to offer them. Often, pharmaceutical drugs have unacceptable side effects. In the case of endometriosis, one problem with some drug therapies is that, while taking them, the woman is infertile because her ovulation is being suppressed by means of pseudomenopause or pseudopregnancy. When she wants to become pregnant, she may find herself caught in a situation where she can't conceive while she has endometriosis, and she can't conceive when she's under treatment for it.

In all forms of healing — allopathic and complementary — much depends on what suits you. Some women will find that a particular pharmaceutical drug works well for them; others will have less success with it. The same occurs with complementary medicine: some women find they respond well to a particular treatment modality, while others have less success with it. Women with endometriosis turn to complementary medicine for a host of reasons. Some try it as a last resort after finding that all available drug and surgical treatments have not resolved the symptoms, while others try it as a first step, before embarking on a course of pharmaceutical drugs or surgery.

Women also have different expectations about what complementary therapies may achieve: some will want to ease particular symptoms; some will want to raise their overall strength or sense of well-being; and others will be aiming for a total cure. Decide what it is you want from complementary therapy, then do some research to find an appropriate modality, and ask around for a practitioner recommended in that field.

Some important considerations:

- Please let your physician know if you intend to follow a complementary medicine route, and give your complementary medicine practitioner full details of your drug regime, if you are on one.
- Your physician or the people at your local health center may be able to refer you to a complementary practitioner they know or work with.
- It is essential with a medical condition like endometriosis to find a therapist who understands the pathology of it and is experienced in treating the condition. Success depends

entirely on the skills of the practitioner you choose. Please ensure that any practitioner you consult has full and proper qualifications in his or her field.

HERBALISM

It's said that a large majority of people in the world today rely on locally grown plants to provide their medicines. The World Health Organization has a long-standing program for the promotion and development of traditional medicines, which they feel can contribute to health care. In more developed areas of the world, the long traditions of local herbalism continue, but with the added benefit of scientific research on the active constituents of particular plants.

Although the word *herbalism* implies that only herbs are used, in fact all types of plants are utilized, but only the particular parts that contain the medicinal value, such as the leaves, roots, petals, stems, seeds, or berries. While many of the plants used in herbalism may seem new to you, some, such as cinnamon or oregano, will be familiar. Both of these are strongly antiviral, and when included in your morning bun or sprinkled on your lunchtime pizza, they actually constitute a form of herbal medicine. In traditional herbalism, plants are chopped up and used as a tea or made into a tincture, which is added to water and drunk. The plant material is also incorporated into creams and lotions for use on the skin, as in, for example, wild yam cream, used as a substitute for hormone replacement therapy. Many herbal remedies are available in capsule form not only from herbalists but also from drugstores, health shops, and supermarkets. Many modern drugs contain active ingredients from plants used in herbalism, and pharmaceutical companies continue to look for new medicinal plants in the rain forests and other remote areas of the world.

At the first consultation, the herbalist will take a full past and present medical history and may ask questions about your lifestyle, diet, exercise, emotional state, and work in order to get a fuller picture of the cause of your problem. This person may also conduct his or her own physical examination.

Herbalism has been found to be effective for skin conditions such as acne, eczema, and psoriasis; allergy problems, including asthma; digestive problems; circulation problems; menstrual problems; stress and anxiety; migraine; chronic fatigue; and arthritis. In the old days, people drank herbal teas because something was wrong — chamomile to aid sleep, fennel for digestive problems, or rosehip as a tonic, for example. These days, however, judging from the number of herbal teas available in supermarkets, cafes, and restaurants, we drink them for pleasure too.

Herbs that may have a beneficial effect on women with endometriosis include agnus castus, peppermint, and milk thistle. More information on these can be found in the self-help treatment program on pages 107–11.

Chinese Herbs

In scientific experiments, several Chinese herbs, including keishi-bukuryo-gan, have demonstrated a beneficial effect in cases of endometriosis and adenomyosis. There are about four hundred Chinese herbs in use, and most of them are roots and fungi rather than the green, leafy plants that the term *herb* may suggest. Most often, Chinese herbs are prescribed as a blend. For example, endometriosis has been successfully treated with a preparation known as "Dan'e Mixture," which is a blend of two roots — *Radix Salviae miltiorrhizae* and *Rhizoma zedoariae*. The first is a copper-colored fibrous root also known as *dan shen*, or "Danshen root." The second is about the same size, but is gray-brown and has the consistency of a hardened, roast chestnut.

Another blend shown to be effective for endometriosis is called Neiyixiao Recipe, which is thought to work by tonifying the kidneys and correcting blood stasis (when there is stoppage or stagnation of blood flow in the vessels). Other herbs might also be chosen because, for example, they "resolve phlegm" or "resolve the lump." Chinese medicine aims to address imbalances so that the proper functioning of all organs is reestablished, leading to health.

Unless you understand Chinese herbs well, it's important to seek the advice of a qualified Chinese herbalist. It is important to be able to identify the herbs, or blend of herbs, being used and to judge their quality. Correct diagnosis is important too. Two very important elements of diagnosis involve the pulse and the tongue, which is examined for color, texture, and coating. A pale tongue might indicate a deficiency in the blood, while a purple tongue indicates stagnation in the liver. Chinese medicine recognizes at least twelve pulses — six in each wrist. The patient's temperature will be taken and face, hands, and body examined. As well as inquiring about physical symptoms, the practitioner may want to know about your emotional life and your home and working environments.

Each herbal mix is put together exclusively for the individual patient. It comes in the form of a dry mix, which you will have to boil to produce a liquid that is drunk like tea.

AYURVEDA

Ayurveda is one of the oldest systems of medicine in the world, one that originated in India perhaps as much as three and a half thousand years ago. It utilizes diet, herbal preparations, massage, steam baths, and yoga exercises. According to Ayurveda, different people who have the same disease may have it for different reasons, and this is why each person is given an individual treatment plan designed to address the basic source of his or her illness. The aim of Ayurveda, as with most other forms of complementary medicine, is to bring the body into balance so it can heal itself. This healing approach recognizes in humans three energy forces (*doshas*) that the Ayurvedic practitioner must balance. These are *vata*, which governs the nervous system and circulation; *kapha*, which governs cellular activity and structures; and *pitta*, which governs metabolism.

The initial consultation will be extensive. The practitioner will record your physical symptoms and collect information about your toilet habits. He or she will also examine your various pulses, your skin, eyes, and tongue, and will try to discover if you are experiencing poor nutrition, digestion, or elimination; if your body or mind is stressed; or if you have lowered immunity, an imbalance of the nervous system, a toxin overload affecting tissues or circulation, or a disturbance of natural rhythms, such as in menstruation or sleep. The Ayurvedic practitioner will be interested in all areas of your life.

Treatment is very likely to begin with a detoxification program, known as *panchakarma*. You may be massaged with herbal oils, which are made by boiling appropriate herbs into a base of vegetable oil — also chosen to correspond to your diagnosis. You may be given an oil to use between treatments and shown how to massage yourself. Certain foods, herbal teas, or yoga positions may be recommended.

In India and Sri Lanka, Ayurvedic students have to study for six years before they can qualify as practitioners. In the West, some people set themselves up as Ayurvedic practitioners after only limited training. Please ensure that any practitioner you consult has full and proper qualifications.

BODYWORK TECHNIQUES, INCLUDING MASSAGE

Bodywork techniques vary widely and range from the gentle stroking, pampering type of massage to the heavy deep-tissue manipulation systems such as Rolfing. Certain bodywork techniques will help you deal with the general tensing of muscles due to constant pain and will stimulate your circulation so your body can activate its own healing potential.

It is extremely important not to subject yourself to vigorous methods of bodywork while you have endometriosis. What you need now is gentle stimulation. Before you make an appointment, make sure the therapist you choose has the appropriate professional training, and inform him or her that you have endometriosis.

The simplest method of bodywork is massage. Often massage practitioners use products that contain essential oils. If you are doing the hip massage outlined in the endometriosis self-help program, take your blend along and ask the therapist to use it on the hip area, in the way outlined. For the rest of the body, a plain organic oil, such as almond, should be used, because the use of essential oils in the program is quite specific, and the addition of other active essential oils may interfere with the path of the regimen.

Some techniques are too physically powerful for women with endometriosis. Although shiatsu, for example, is often described as a gentle therapy, it can be extremely physical. Rolfing is another therapy that can be rough on the body, and it should perhaps be avoided for the time being. Rolfing aligns the body by manipulating the muscles, fascia, and connective tissue, and the touch may feel too intense, particularly if you have scar tissue.

People have been massaging each other since time began — to relieve pain or just for pleasure. Around the world, different systems of massage have developed, including Swedish, Indian, Indonesian, Japanese, Chinese, Thai, Turkish, and Hawaiian. In many countries, massage is part of everyday life, and mothers massage their babies, and grandmothers get pain-relieving joint-massages from attentive family members. The Western world has become less hands-on, as we rely more on medical drugs to cure our stress and our muscle pain. However, modern medicine has started to embrace the benefits that massage can bring, especially in preventive health care and convalescence.

The ancients were very clear about the benefits of massage. Hippocrates, the Greek "father of medicine," wrote, "The way to health is to have a scented bath and an oiled massage daily," and the Romans continued the tradition in their famous bathhouses. The art of massage was lost to Western society for many years but was revived in the nineteenth century by the Swedish sportsman and intellectual Per Henrik Ling. Today his system of Swedish massage is the starting point for many types of bodywork, although it's been joined in popularity by many other systems, including lymphatic therapy, connective tissue manipulation, Hellerwork, Marma, Indian head massage, and body harmonics — the latter is a combination of the Thai, Chinese, and Indonesian traditions.

Massage is the manipulation of the skin and underlying flesh and is thought to help stimulate the elimination of toxins from the body. Because massage is mostly done directly on the skin, usually using some form of lubricant like oil, cream, or talc, you'll be asked to remove most of your clothing, depending on which areas are to be massaged. The therapist will place a towel over the part of your body not being worked on. The room should be warm and free of drafts.

There are innumerable systems of massage. Two of the most popular are Swedish massage and lymphatic therapy. Swedish massage incorporates the movements known as effleurage (stroking), petrissage (kneading), friction (pressure), and percussion (drumming with closed fists). Lymphatic therapy incorporates work on the lymphatic system, in which toxins can accumulate. "Lymphatic drainage" can be a good treatment for someone with edema, or water retention, as well as for a person with recurring colds and flu.

Experienced bodyworkers use their hands as a communication system and as a diagnostic tool. The skill and art of massage entails rhythmically unraveling the story the body has to tell, through touching the knotted muscles, exploring the stiffness and tension, allowing the body to rebalance and harmonize.

Above all, massage is an effective form of stress relief. It increases circulation and, because of this, the flow of oxygen throughout the body. It can help specific areas of muscle pain, keep the body supple and free of stiffness, and act as a general tonifier.

ACUPUNCTURE AND ACUPRESSURE

Acupuncture is an integral part of Chinese medicine, in which an acupuncturist places extremely fine stainless steel needles into the skin and leaves them there for around thirty minutes. Although the scientific basis of acupuncture is not known, Western doctors have been amazed to observe serious surgical procedures carried out at the famous Beijing Acupuncture and Anesthesia Clinic in which no anesthesia other than acupuncture was used, and have brought acupuncture into mainstream medicine.

Acupuncture is known to be thousands of years old, and there are said to be over three million practitioners around the world today. Their aim, simply put, is to restore balance to the body so it can heal itself. This treatment approach is based on an energy, chi, that flows throughout the body but most particularly in twelve energy channels, known as meridians. An imbalance in this energy flow can be caused by many things, such as infection, toxins, poor diet, trauma, weather conditions, hereditary factors, and emotional states, including grief, anger, fear, and stress.

To bring the flow of chi into balance, the acupuncturist places needles in precise points along the meridians. There are more than a thousand acupuncture points on the body, but a treatment usually involves between six and twelve points. Common places for needle insertion are the shoulders, back, abdomen, feet, hands, and ears. The needles are often used in points that are a long way away from the site of the problem.

In China, acupuncture is accompanied by herbal medicine, especially moxibustion — which is the setting alight of an herb, Artemesia vulgaris (mugwort). The smoldering herb is placed on top of the needle, or an herb-cone is placed over the acupuncture site. Sometimes just the smoke of the herb is wafted over the area. There are now additional modern techniques in acupuncture. Some acupuncturists stimulate the needles electrically by clipping electrodes to them, which vibrate the needles. Laser acupuncture is a newer adaptation.

Before the first session, the acupuncturist may ask many questions. These will cover your past and present medical history, emotional state, sleep patterns, and bodily functions, such as digestion. The color, structure, and coating of your tongue may be examined.

Another important aspect of the consultation involves taking your pulse. Chinese medicine recognizes twelve pulses — six in each wrist — which are related to the twelve meridians. The acupuncturist will measure not only the rhythm of each pulse but also its strength and "quality." You will need to remove clothing only in the areas of the body where the acupuncturist intends to insert needles. There is a slight sensation when the needles go in, but it's nothing like an injection. After treatment, in some cases, there can be a little bruising, but it shouldn't be painful. Acupuncture is said to be good for pain relief, muscle spasm, asthma, hay fever, and male and female reproductive problems. It can be used simultaneously with Western drugs.

Acupressure is the system of applying pressure to the meridian points with the fingers rather than with needles. The basic goal is the same — to rebalance the body by stimulating the flow of chi. This therapy is less regulated than acupuncture, and it is often incorporated into other healing modalities, such as massage.

HYDROTHERAPY

Hydrotherapy is a term that covers a lot of different practices, all involving water. In a sense, having a warm bath is hydrotherapy because it's relaxing and calming. Hot water increases circulation of both blood and lymph and contributes to the elimination of toxins. Cold water is essential in controlling a fever, is useful in cases of inflammation, and is a form of stimulating hydrotherapy because it perks you up. Some treatments use alternating hot and cold water. Alternating between the two temperature extremes stimulates the functioning of the body, including that of the organs. Heat dilates blood vessels, while cold constricts them. The body starts working more efficiently, less sluggishly, which contributes to the healing process.

There are different forms of hydrotherapy practiced around the world, especially where there are mineral springs. Some healing systems use water therapies combined with herbs, as in Ayurvedic baths, for example, or essential oils, as in aromatherapy.

Three different components define the particular branches of hydrotherapy: the method, which includes whether the water is applied as a liquid, as steam, or in solid form, as ice; the temperature of the water; and any additions to the water such as minerals, salts, and seaweed.

The practice of hydrotherapy incorporates the following methods.

- Hosing: The therapist aims a powerful jet of water at your body. This method is used in European health spas to increase circulation and break down cellulite. It can be quite painful and is not recommended for women with endometriosis, because too much force might be applied to affected areas of the body.
- Underwater massage: This method is usually used on people with chronic pain, especially those with immobile joints or limbs, because the tissue is supported by the water.
- Underwater exercise: This is particularly good for those who have weak or wasted muscles as a result of underuse. It is also an excellent form of gentle exercise for women with endometriosis.
- Ice and water: Wrapped bags of ice are placed on painful areas to help reduce inflammation. Bags of frozen peas are equally effective.
- Cold compresses: These can be used to reduce inflammation.
- Hot compresses: These increase blood flow to diseased or injured parts or organs of the body.
- Sitz baths: Sitz baths are an important component of the endometriosis self-help treatment program (see page 83).

Do not use hydrotherapy if you suffer from high blood pressure or if you have a heart condition. Water can adversely affect some people if it is too hot or too cold, or if the change from hot water to cold, or vice versa, is too quick. Dizziness or fainting can occur.

HOMEOPATHY

Homeopathy was invented around 1810 by a German physician, Samuel Hahnemann. He discovered that an herbal remedy for malaria, cinchona tree bark (which contains quinine), caused the symptoms of malaria when taken in excess by a healthy person. This led him to believe that substances that cause symptoms similar to those of a particular disease could possibly be used to treat it. "Homeopathy" means "like-disease," and homeopaths often use the expression "like cures like" to explain it. Treatment is given in the form of tinctures, tablets, granules, powders, and skin creams.

There are more than two thousand homeopathic remedies, and the raw material for them is extremely diverse, including plants and minerals but also some substances that are much less attractive sounding. If you use homeopathic remedies, find out which material each remedy has been derived from.

We're told that these raw materials do not in themselves remain in the remedies, and that the stage of their preparation known as succussion — vigorous shaking — imprints the unique energy pattern of the raw material onto the water in which it's diluted, so there's no need for the material itself to remain.

The more diluted the remedy, the more potent it is said to be. This confounds scientists, who can't understand how homeopathy can possibly work. The Society of Homeopaths in the United Kingdom says the answer to this puzzling question "is likely to be found outside the chemistry laboratory in the field of physics, especially electro-magnetism." As it is not the chemistry of the remedy that causes change in the body, but rather the energy of the material, it is only necessary to introduce the vibration of the remedy rather than detectable chemical substances. For this reason, homeopathic preparations are in a sense substance free and seem to be extremely safe.

The first appointment with a homeopath can take between half an hour and an hour. Subsequent visits may take less time. Homeopaths not only take a full medical history but also ask questions such as "Do you prefer sweet or salty foods?" "Do you like the mountains or the sea?" or "Do you feel better in hot or cold weather?" Many of their questions may seem irrelevant to your health problem, but your answers help the homeopath build up a picture of what kind of person you are and decide which remedy to prescribe.

Endometriosis is a chronic condition that has deep-seated causes and requires what is known as a "constitutional remedy." The condition also involves symptoms that come and go, particularly at different times of the menstrual cycle, and these may require an "acute remedy." Homeopathy is a complex subject, and you'll likely have the best results if you consult with a qualified professional rather than attempt to treat yourself, especially with a chronic condition like endometriosis. That said, the following is a list of some of the remedies that might be recommended for endometriosis.

Calcarea:
Pain on the left side of the uterus or groin before or during menstruation; discharge; lower back pain; general unwellness.

Sepia:
Premenstrual syndrome; painful menstruation or intercourse; anger.

Lachesis:
Premenstrual pain in either the lower abdomen or the left ovary; jealousy.

Lilium tigrum:
Pain in the ovaries, spreading to the upper thighs; weepiness; anxiousness.

Colocynthis:
Cramp pain that lessens when you double over; premenstrual anger.

Belladona:
Sudden onset of intense cramps or other pain, spreading to the legs; pain lessens when you straighten your body; hot flashes; bright red and profuse blood flow; sensitivity to touch and movement.

Other homeopathic remedies that might be recommended are chamomilla, china, graphites, platina, nux vomica, phosphorus, pulsatilla, and veratrum alb. Homeopathic remedies are available in pharmacies and health stores and are prescribed by homeopathic specialists, some of whom are also medical doctors.

BIOCHEMIC CELL SALTS

The system known as "biochemic cell salts" focuses on the body's need for certain minerals, such as calcium, chlorine, magnesium, phosphorus, potassium, sodium, and sulfur; trace minerals (microminerals), such as iron and fluoride; and certain elements, such as silicon.

The body needs minerals to function correctly. For example, muscle contraction and the transmission of nerve impulses rely on sufficient calcium, potassium, sodium, magnesium, and phosphorus; sulfur is a crucial constituent of certain proteins, including insulin.

The cell salts are prepared in the homeopathic way: the mineral salt is repeatedly diluted with lactose. However, they differ from homeopathic preparations in that they aim to replace deficiencies in the cells. The homeopathic method of preparation allows for the tiniest of amounts to be taken.

With modern farming methods, especially monoculture, many of the natural nutrients once found in the ground and absorbed by the plant material available to us as food have been lost. You know your own eating habits and symptoms, and you should research this subject further if you intend to use these interesting preparations.

There are twelve main biochemic cell salts and thirty minor ones. The components of the cell salts were devised by the German physician Wilhelm Schuessler in 1873. Up to three cell salts may be taken at the same time.

A recommended combination for pain during menstruation is Ferr Phos and Kali Mur. For women who have been on long drug therapy routines, a combination of Nat Mur and Kali Sulph is a good option for clearing the body of toxins. Maintain the routine for two weeks.

Follow the instructions on the packaging. Each dose may consist of up to four tablets. If you are using two cell salts at the same time, it's often recommended to take them alternately — that is, take one tissue salt in the morning, the other two hours later, the first two hours after that, and so on until you have taken three doses of each over the course of the day.

The twelve main biochemic cell salts are listed below, along with the symptoms that they address. Look at the box for each, and decide which one addresses the largest number of your symptoms.

The Twelve Main Biochemic Cell Salts

---

1. Calcarea Fluorica (from calcium flouride)

Chemical formula: CaF_2

Shortened name: Calc Fluor

Primary focus in the body: Tissue elasticity

Symptoms addressed:

- Profuse menstrual flow
- Menstruation with "bearing down" pain
- Pain extending down the thighs
- Dragging pain in the groin area
- General back pain
- Lower back pain with a dragging sensation
- Leg pain, with a sensation of heaviness
- Anal itching, fissures, hemorrhoids; difficulty passing stools

2. Calcarea Phosphorica (from calcium phosphate)

Chemical formula: $Ca_3(PO_4)_2$

Shortened name: Calc Phos

Primary focus in the body: Nutrition

Symptoms addressed:

- Menstrual cycle is too short
- Cold hands and feet during menstruation
- Painful uterine cramps
- Dull ache in the uterus
- Back pain during menstruation
- Flushed face during menstruation
- Bone and joint pains, especially at night

3. Calcarea Sulphurica (from calcium sulfate)

Chemical formula: $CaSO_4\ 12H_2O$

Shortened name: Calc Sulph

Primary focus in the body: Detoxification and healing

Symptoms addressed:

- Thick discharge from the vagina

4. Ferrum Phosphoricum (from iron phosphate)

Chemical formula: $Fe(PO_4)_2$

Shortened name: Ferr Phos

Primary focus in the body: Oxygenation

Symptoms addressed:

- Painful periods with congestion (dysmenorrhea)
- Cold hands and feet during menstruation
- Headache during menstruation
- Bright red menstrual flow
- Nausea or vomiting
- Inflammation in the abdomen
- Cutting pains in the abdomen
- Pain (anywhere) that throbs, feels inflamed and congested

5. Chloride of Potassium (from potassium chloride)

Chemical formula: KC1

Shortened name: Kali Mur

Primary focus in the body: Blood cleansing

Symptoms addressed:

- Menstrual cycles last less than twenty-eight days; lengthy menstrual flow
- Heavy menstrual flow
- Menstrual flow is infrequent
- Blood is dark and clotted
- Swollen abdomen
- Pain in the liver area or under the right shoulder blade
- Slow metabolism

6. *Kali Phosphoricum (from potassium phosphate)*

Chemical formula: K_2HPO_4

Shortened name: Kali Phos

Primary focus in the body: Nerves

Symptoms addressed:

- Menstruation is delayed
- Menstrual flow is dark red
- Headache during menstruation
- Nervousness during menstruation
- Menstrual flow is heavy
- Menstrual flow is thin and watery
- Swollen abdomen
- Left-side pain in the abdomen, with flatulence

7. *Kali Sulphuricum (from potassium sulfate)*

Chemical formula: K_2SO_4

Shortened name: Kali Sulph

Primary focus in the body: Respiration

Symptoms addressed:

- Abdomen feels swollen or heavy during menstruation
- Menstruation is delayed
- Bloating in the abdomen
- Painful twinges in the abdomen, possibly moving position

8. Magnesia Phosphorica (from magnesium phosphate)

Chemical formula: $MgHPO_47H_2O$

Shortened name: Mag Phos

Primary focus in the body: Spasms

Symptoms addressed:

- Severe abdominal cramps, possibly with heavy menstrual flow
- Menstrual flow stringlike and thickened
- Intestinal cramps during menstruation
- Premenstrual abdominal pain
- Ovarian pain
- Flatulence with sulfurous odor
- Pain (anywhere) is accompanied by spasm or cramping
- Pain (anywhere) is sharp or knifelike

9. Natrium Muriaticum (from sodium chloride — common salt)

Chemical formula: NaC1

Shortened name: Nat Mur

Primary focus in the body: Waste distribution

Symptoms addressed:

- Headache during menstruation
- Sadness and weeping during menstruation
- Thin, watery menstrual flow
- Discharge causing pain to mucous membrane of vagina and labia
- Pain to mucous membrane of vagina and labia after urination
- Dry vagina
- Burning pain in the rectum
- Swollen abdomen with flatulence

10. *Natrium Phosphoricum (from sodium phosphate)*

Chemical formula: $Na_2HPO_412H_2O$

Shortened name: Nat Phos

Primary focus in the body: Acid neutralization

Symptoms addressed:

- Creamy discharge from the vagina
- Itchy anus

11. *Natrium Sulphuricum (from sodium sulfate)*

Chemical formula: Na_2SO_4

Shortened name: Nat Sulph

Primary focus in the body: Liver and kidneys

Symptoms addressed:

- Intestinal cramps during menstruation
- Constipation during menstruation
- Morning diarrhea during menstruation
- Intestinal pain with flatulence

12. *Silicea (from silicon dioxide)*

Chemical formula: SiO_2

Shortened name: Silicea

Primary focus in the body: Cleansing and elimination

Symptoms addressed:

- Heavy flow during menstruation
- Constipation during menstruation
- Body feels cold during menstruation

FLOWER REMEDIES

Flower remedies have become very popular, and there seem to be more and more different types available each year. There are New Zealand, Californian, Alaskan, and Hawaiian flower remedies, and Australian bush remedies, and many more. It seems there isn't a corner of the globe that isn't now producing its own version of the original flower remedies, created in the 1930s by the London physician Edward Bach.

Dr. Bach discovered that certain plants, when left in water in the sun, produced a tincture that helped people rebalance and overcome particular negative emotional states. The raw materials of his remedies were plants growing around his country cottage in Oxfordshire. There are thirty-eight remedies in total, plus a "rescue remedy," which is the most popular of the Bach preparations.

There are several ways to take the prepared remedies. Usually four drops are put in a glass of water, which is sipped throughout the day. Two or more remedies can be used together.

Dr. Bach's thirty-eight remedies are arranged in seven broad groupings; see the table "Bach Flower Remedies."

BACH FLOWER REMEDIES

Symptom	Recommended Remedy
Fear	
Terror	Rock Rose
Fear of known things	Mimulus
Fear of mental breakdown	Cherry plum
Fears and worries of unknown origin	Aspen
Fear or overconcern for others	Red chestnut
Loneliness	
Pride, aloofness	Water violet
Impatience	Impatiens
Self-centeredness, self-concern	Heather
Insufficient Interest in Present Circumstances	
Dreaminess, lack of interest in present	Clematis
Tendency to live in the past	Honeysuckle
Resignation, apathy	Wild rose
Lack of energy	Olive
Unwanted thoughts, mental arguments	White chestnut
Deep gloom with no origin	Mustard
Failure to learn from past mistakes	Chestnut bud
Despondency or Despair	
Lack of confidence	Larch
Self-reproach, guilt	Pine
Tendency to feel overwhelmed by responsibility	Elm
Extreme mental anguish	Sweet chestnut
Aftereffects of shock	Star of Bethlehem
Resentment	Willow
Exhaustion while one struggles on	Oak
Self-hatred, sense of uncleanliness	Crab apple

(Continued on next page)

BACH FLOWER REMEDIES (*CONTINUED*)

Symptom	Recommended Remedy
Uncertainty	
Tendency to seek advice and confirmation from others	Cerato
Indecision	Scleranthus
Discouragement, despondency	Gentian
Hopelessness and despair	Gorse
"Monday morning" feeling	Hornbeam
Uncertainty about the correct path in life	Wild oat
Oversensitivity to Influences and Ideas	
Mental torment behind a brave face	Agrimony
Weak will, subservience	Centaury
Protection from change and outside influences	Walnut
Hatred, envy, jealousy	Holly
Overcare for the Welfare of Others	
Selfish possessiveness	Chicory
Overenthusiasm	Vervain
Domination, inflexibility	Vine
Intolerance	Beech
Self-repression, self-denial	Rock water

Dr. Bach designed the flower remedies as a self-help system. They are safe to use, although you must bear in mind that these, and indeed most, flower remedies are preserved in alcohol.

NATUROPATHY

Naturopathy, or naturopathic medicine, is quintessentially holistic. It is an all-encompassing healing modality, one that draws on all branches of complementary medicine to achieve its goals. Naturopathy has three guiding principles:

- The body has the power to heal itself.
- The methods used must be gentle, efficient, and as noninvasive as possible.
- The healer must look for and treat the cause of the problem rather than the symptoms.

Naturopathy uses every available helpful tool to achieve its goal of stimulating the body into healing itself. Because naturopathy fully recognizes the mind-body connection, the naturopath may recommend counseling and stress management techniques, as well as breathing exercises, physical exercise, stretching techniques, physical therapy, yoga, tai chi, chi gong, or hydrotherapy. Manipulation of both bones and soft tissue is often incorporated into treatment in the form of massage, osteopathy, or chiropractic. In addition, the naturopath might recommend homeopathy or herbal medicine, and dietary changes or nutritional supplementation.

Because each person is an individual, each person receives individual treatment tailored to his or her particular symptoms, lifestyle, posture, exercise routine, mental attitude, and diet. The naturopath truly sees people "in the round" — holistically. The practitioner will want to know about your stress levels, as stress can suppress the immune system, for example, and about your work pattern, as overwork can put particular strains on the body.

With all these aspects to consider and potential treatment modalities to learn about, a naturopath requires a fair amount of training time. A fully qualified naturopath spends many years in full-time naturopathic education, during which he or she learns many different skills, including body manipulation techniques, for example. However, the naturopath may recommend that you go to a specialist in a particular field of complementary medicine for additional treatment. Because naturopathy involves so many branches of complementary medicine, most naturopaths are on an unending path of education to continually broaden their knowledge base and skills. Some naturopaths are additionally trained in conventional diagnostic procedures such as X-ray and laboratory testing.

Someone who has undergone a full course of training can be called a Doctor of Naturopathy, and it is this level of proficiency that a woman with endometriosis must seek in the practitioner she chooses. Many fully qualified naturopaths work in an integrated way with physicians, and it would be wise to ask your general practitioner if he or she can recommend a naturopath to you. A women with endometriosis should try to avoid taking professional advice from someone who has completed only a short course in the subject. Naturopathy involves so many aspects of healing that it simply cannot be learned in a short time. Be sure that the practitioner you consult is fully licensed.

On the first visit, the naturopath will want to know all about you. Your diet, work and relationship details, health record, and posture will be among the things noted. He or she will record your blood pressure, check your pulse, or arrange for collecting further information in the form of X-rays or blood or urine samples. Although the naturopath may carry out some form of physical manipulation and assess where changes are needed, you are the one who must make those changes. For this reason, naturopathy is about taking responsibility for your own treatment, with the naturopath acting as a teacher, guide, and supporter.

PART THREE

Supporting Information

CHAPTER NINE

Essential Oils

Essential oils are concentrated plant essences that form in specialized cells of certain plants. Depending on the plant species, the essential oil is produced in the leaves, flowers, seeds, stalks, twigs, bark, wood, or roots. In some plants, such as marjoram, the oil forms in all parts of the plant, and in others it forms in very particular places, such as in the resin exuding from the bark of a tree.

Different methods are used to extract the essential oil from the plant material. The most common are steam and water distillation. About three hundred essential oils are used by the perfumery and cosmetics trade, the food and drinks industries, the pharmaceutical industry, and holistic therapies such as aromatherapy. The term *oil* is somewhat misleading, because, depending on the species from which it was distilled, the essential oil is more likely to be watery, viscous, or even semisolid.

The molecules that create the strong aromas of essential oils are volatile: they evaporate. Some essential oils, such as those from the citrus group — for example, orange, lemon, lime, and grapefruit, whose oils are extracted from the peel — tend to evaporate more quickly than others.

Many familiar culinary herbs contain essential oils, including basil, oregano, rosemary, sage, thyme, coriander, marjoram, and tarragon, as do spices, such as ginger, cinnamon, cardamom, and clove. Other essential oils come from plants so delightful that people have nurtured them in their gardens for at least as long as historical records have been kept, such as in the case of rose and jasmine. Others come from shrubs or trees in the form of resins that exude like pearls from the bark, inviting us to harvest them. These include frankincense and myrrh, which have long been valued for producing aromas suitable to religious practice. The invigorating aroma of a pine forest derives from the essential oils stored in the pines' thin needles. Generations have sipped peppermint, chamomile, and other herbal teas recognized for their medicinal value. In these and other ways, human beings have been coevolving with the plants that yield essential oils. They have been part of our daily lives and are woven into our history.

THE IMPORTANCE OF PURITY

A woman following the endometriosis self-help program will require five or six essential oils. The purity of each one is crucial to the success of the program. Aim to purchase essential oils that are organic or "wild crafted" — a term indicating that they have been carefully collected from the wild.

The human nose is still the most effective tool for determining the quality of an essential oil, according to people working to establish oil purity. This is good to know because it is difficult for consumers to ensure that the essential oils on sale have the qualities stated in the marketing material or on the packaging. This is despite advances in technology to determine the various characteristic markers of pure, good-quality essential oils.

The best way to determine the quality of essential oils is to educate yourself about the different aromas and practical qualities of oils from different suppliers. Make a point of going into shops and trying out the testers of the essential oils on sale there. Become familiar with differences in aroma between all the brands, using two or three oils as your standard. That is, always smell the same "tester" essential oils. A broad range of oils to use as your sample could be lavender, which is light; neroli, which is slightly thicker; and patchouli, which is viscous. Get to know how they smell. Read the literature, get a feel for suppliers' attitudes toward the customer.

THE COMPLEX WORLD OF ESSENTIAL OILS

Plant species produce varying amounts of essential oil. For example, it takes between 3,000 and 4,000 pounds of hand-picked roses to produce only 1 pound of rose oil, while it takes only 5 pounds of cloves to yield approximately 1 pound of clove essential oil. Not surprisingly, rose is expensive, and clove is not.

Some essential oils have a very short aromatic and/or therapeutic life, while others last longer. The citrus oils are best used fresh, while others — such as patchouli, sandalwood, jasmine, benzoin, and myrrh — improve with age.

Essential oils are still somewhat mysterious compounds. In rose oil (*Rosa damascena*), the main chemical constituents — including citronellol, geraniol, nerol, and stearopten — may represent around 86 percent of the volume, and another 300 compounds could make up the other 14 percent. Those substances, tiny though their relative volume may be, make rose oil what it is: more than a collection of a few chemicals.

Some essential oils — such as tea tree, citronella, and sweet orange — are seldom adulterated because they are cheaper than the adulterant itself. Other essential oils escape adulteration because their major chemical components — usually the added adulterants — are difficult to obtain. Vetiver and patchouli essential oils often fall into this group.

If you are buying essential oils to heat in diffusers, their 100 percent chemical assurance would not be vital. But, when you use essential oils for body or facial therapy, and the essential oils are being absorbed by the skin, it is crucial to know that they are 100 percent pure and have the intended therapeutic ability.

Among different samples of an essential oil — lavender, for example — there is wide variation in aroma and therapeutic quality, which results from differences in the geographic locations where the lavender plants were grown. For example, the same species of lavender would have a somewhat different chemical profile and therapeutic effect — depending on static elements such as the altitude and nutrient profile of the soil — when grown in a different location. The weather conditions in any given year also have a huge impact on the character of any individual essential oil, and these conditions include the number of sunny days, volume of rainfall, temperature levels, amount of wind, and the presence of frost. Annual crops especially have good years and bad years, like wine. Variation may occur in aroma, chemical profile, and therapeutic effect, as well as in yield. Even the time of day that the crop is harvested can make an enormous difference in the volume and quality of essential oil produced, as can the length of time the crop material is exposed to the distillation process.

All these variables can create somewhat different essential oils even from the same crop, but all the resulting samples will be variations of a natural, 100 percent pure essential oil extracted from a particular named species — and this is the definition of a good essential oil.

When there ceases to be variation in essential oils, it suggests that the oils may have been adulterated to make them conform to some standard required by the main industrial users of essential oils — the perfumery trade and the food and drink industries. Industry likes to know that the ingredients it uses are consistent, even if this means turning a blind eye when producers mix in a few extra chemical compounds now and again. And because the main focus of industry is cost, producers may be tempted to extend their product by adding other, cheaper materials. They may also add chemical constituents in an attempt to pass off a poor-quality or badly distilled essential oil as one of a better quality. Adulteration methods include

- mixing an essential oil with cheaper versions of the same essential oil species;
- mixing it with a cheaper essential oil of a different species but with a similar aroma;
- adding a cheaper natural product, such as rapeseed oil, that cannot be detected by gas chromatography;
- adding a cheaper chemical product, such as benzyl alcohol, that can be detected by gas chromatography;
- adding perfume bases to bulk up the thicker essential oils;
- distilling with cheaper essential oil plant materials of another species.

The most sought-after geranium essential oil, for example, is known as "Bourbon," and it comes from Réunion, an island near Madagascar. But the demand for it outstrips supply, so unscrupulous producers take Chinese geranium oil and try to give it the chemical profile of the more expensive Bourbon geranium oil by adding specific synthetic or natural chemicals.

There are many tests available that together build a physiochemical profile of an essential oil and measure its quality. The tests determine whether a given essential oil has the known, and expected, characteristics of that species. The tests include gas chromatography, which assesses whether the major chemical compounds and trace elements characteristic of each oil are present, in the correct ratio, and for the specific chemicals found in adulterant materials.

In addition, gas chromatography combined with mass spectrography assesses components in terms of their molecular mass spectrum.

Tests for specific gravity compare the weight of the essential oil to an equal volume of water. The refractive index of an essential oil measures the refraction of light when passed through it: if the angle of refraction does not fall within the expected range for the particular essential oil species, this can indicate that it's been adulterated or is of low quality. Tests for optical rotation involve passing a beam of polarized light through the essential oil sample. If the light is bent to the left, or in a counterclockwise direction, it is said to be levorotatory; and, if bent to the right or clockwise direction, it is dextrorotatory. Each essential oil is expected to react in a certain way if it is pure, and it is this that is being tested.

There are other tests to establish the various qualities of essential oils, and more are being developed all the time. However, while these tests can help establish the components in a given oil, they do not tell us whether the essential oil has residues of pesticides, herbicides, fungicides, dioxins, and heavy metals. The best way to ensure the quality of an essential oil is to buy organic.

CHOOSING ORGANICALLY GROWN OILS

The best essential oils to use in the endometriosis self-help program are organic or wild crafted. Essential oils derived from organically grown plants are those distilled from plant material cultivated without chemically synthesized insecticides, herbicides, fungicides, or other pesticides. Essential oils derived from wild crafted plants are those distilled from plant material that has been harvested in a sustainable fashion from trees and other plants that grow wild in a certain region. These are essentially organic, in the sense that they have not been treated with chemicals. Examples of these include cedarwood, cypress, eucalyptus, frankincense, rosemary, thyme, and marjoram. If the bottle says "wild crafted," then the oil is as pure as those labeled "organic."

Not all suppliers label their products as "organic" or "wild crafted" even when they are. And just because an essential oil is not labeled as either "wild crafted" or "organic," it doesn't mean that the oil is not natural. Many companies sell fine essential oils derived from plant material grown organically by farmers or growers not registered with the local organic certification authority. Fees can often be expensive in some countries and may cost more than poorer farmers can afford. The best solution is to ask the supplier of the essential oil.

Each country has its own regulations regarding the accepted classification of organic produce, as well as organizations that oversee the certification of these products. In general, they do not allow growers to use synthetic pesticides or fertilizers, but do allow the use of a few natural pesticides. And, with the organic system of farming, fertilization of the soil may be accomplished by means of compost and other natural materials (which must themselves be organic). However, an essential oil purportedly from an organic source may not have been tested for the presence of chemical pesticides and fertilizers because, while the soil is tested by the regulating organization, the product itself is not.

KNOWLEDGE IS POWER

The purity of essential oils is important to everyone who uses them, including the food, drink, and pharmaceutical industries. Another main user is the cosmetics and perfumery trade, and it was in a research and development lab associated with this industry where Dr. Shizuo Torii and colleagues analyzed the relative ratios of the main constituents in lavender and tea tree essential oils. They determined that the variation in the chemical constituents of these essential oils was too broad and recommended that quality control by means of instrumental analysis be more widely introduced, and that the results be made available to the public.

As more information is built up, and as improvements in

technology enable researchers to identify more of the trace elements in essential oils, the databases should expand to include some of the wider variations between species. For example, at present the *French Pharmacopeia* states that the amount of linalyl acetate esters (a natural component of lavender oil) to be expected in *Lavender officinalis* is between 35 and 55 percent. However, some of the best French lavender is cultivated fourteen hundred meters above sea level, in the Haute Provence region, and contains up to 70 percent. This higher ester content occurs not only because this wild-growing lavender contains more natural linalyl esters but also because, at such high altitude, the temperature required for distillation falls from 100 degrees centigrade to 93. The lavender oil distilled from these plants is of higher medicinal value and can be produced only at high altitude, and yet it does not fall inside the "normal" parameters established at sea-level distillation plants. So, although it is an excellent essential oil, it is not certified as organic. Such anomalies in the present certification system should be ironed out as time goes on, and as the reference databases used in testing incorporate a wider range of information about essential oils.

For all the reasons above, it is important to choose your essential oil supplier carefully. Use a specialist supplier rather than purchasing from supermarkets or drugstores. A good supplier will be able to tell you from which part of the plant the oil is distilled, in which country it was grown, and its botanical name. Such a supplier will also be able to tell you whether the plant material was wild crafted or cultivated and whether it is organic. If neither organic nor wild crafted essential oils are available, use essential oils that are marked "100 percent natural essential oil." This should ensure that the plant material has not been adulterated with any other substance.

SAFETY NOTES CONCERNING ESSENTIAL OILS

There are some basic rules to remember when using essential oils — whether undiluted or diluted:

- Never take them internally, orally, unless under specific professional guidance.
- Avoid getting essential oils near the eyes.
- Some essential oils increase the photosensitivity of the skin, and they should not be used before going out in the sun, or into a solarium, or before using a sunbed. This applies to essential oils used either diluted or undiluted, and whether applied to the face or body. These photosensitive oils include bergamot, lemon, lime, orange, mandarin, tangerine, clementine, grapefruit, angelica root, and yarrow.
- Before using any particular essential oil, check its contraindications to ensure that none apply to you.
- If you are taking prescribed medication, consult your physician before commencing any form of complementary or alternative regime.
- Keep essential oils and blends away from children.
- Store essential oils and blends in a cool, dark, dry place.

ESSENTIAL OILS USED IN THE CORE ENDOMETRIOSIS NATURAL TREATMENT PROGRAM

Bergamot

Latin name: *Citrus aurantium* ssp. *bergamia*

Plant family: Rutaceae

Type of plant: Tree with white star-shaped flowers and small green citrus fruit

Part used: Rind of both ripe and unripe fruit

Method of extraction: Cold expression

Country of production: 90 percent of the world's crop is produced in the Reggio di Calabria region of Italy.

When buying, look for: A greenish yellow watery liquid with a fruity, fresh citrus aroma and spicy floral undertones.

Bergamot is the main flavoring in Earl Grey tea. It's also widely used in eau de cologne. It was named after the northern Italian town of Bergamo but is now mainly produced in Calabria, in southern Italy. The green tint of bergamot oil results from the chlorophyll content.

An annual herb also called bergamot (*Monarda didyma*) has no relation to the bergamot used in essential oil.

Caution or Contraindications: Bergamot contains bergaptene, which is phototoxic — that is, it amplifies the effect of sunlight. Bergamot should not be applied to the skin — even in diluted form — or used in the bath, before exposure to the sun or a sunbed. A bergaptene-free bergamot (bergamot FCF) is available.

Chamomile Roman

Latin name: *Anthemis nobilis*

Plant family: Asteraceae

Type of plant: Small plant with feathery leaves and small white flowers

Part used: Flowers and leaves

Method of extraction: Steam distillation

Countries of production: England, Bulgaria, Hungary, Chile, France

When buying, look for: A clear, watery liquid, with a slight blue-green tinge and a fruity, sweet, fresh, herbal, applelike aroma

For over two thousand years, chamomile has been used extensively as a medicine. The Latin name derives from the Greek *anthemis*, meaning "little flower." In ancient Egyptian and early Scandinavian cultures, chamomile was associated with the sun god.

Caution or Contraindications: None known.

Clary Sage

Latin name: *Salvia sclarea*

Plant family: Lamiaceae (Labiatae)

Type of plant: Biennial plant with large hairy leaves and lilac-pink flowers

Part used: Flowering tops

Method of extraction: Steam distillation

Countries of production: France, Bulgaria, Russia, England, Germany

When buying, look for: A watery, colorless or pale yellow liquid with a nutty, warm, light, musky, herbaceous aroma

The term *salvia* is derived from the Latin for "good health." The seeds have been used in many countries to clear conditions of the eye — hence its common name, "clear-eye." In Germany the herb was used, along with elderflowers, as an additive to cheap wine to make it taste like muscatel.

Caution or Contraindications: Avoid during pregnancy.

Cypress

Latin name: *Cupressus sempervirens*

Plant family: Cupressaceae

Type of plant: Evergreen tree with dark-green foliage

Part used: Foliage and twigs

Method of extraction: Steam distillation

Countries of production: France, Spain

When buying, look for: A colorless to slightly yellow, watery liquid with a woody, warm, slightly spicy aroma

The tree gave its name to the island of Cyprus. Due to the essential oil content, the wood of this tree is impervious to woodworms, making it especially useful for works of art and furniture. Cypress essential oil is a common ingredient in men's colognes.

Caution or Contraindications: None known.

Fennel (Sweet)

Latin name: *Foeniculum vulgare dulce*

Plant family: Apiaceae (Umbelliferae)

Type of plant: Tall biennial herb growing up to five feet, with delicate, feathery, lacelike leaves and small yellow flowers on a flowering head

Part used: Seeds

Method of extraction: Steam distillation

Countries of production: Bulgaria, Hungary, France, Germany, Italy, India

When buying, look for: A colorless to pale yellow watery liquid with a warm, sweet, aniseedlike, peppery aroma

Fennel was a favorite with the ancient Greeks and Romans, who used it extensively in medicine and cooking. They believed it gave strength and long life, and helped the eyesight, lactation, menstrual problems, and a great deal besides. Fishermen first understood its taste affinity with fish, possibly because fennel often grows near the coast.

Caution or Contraindications: Not to be used during pregnancy or while breastfeeding, or by people with epilepsy.

Geranium

Latin name: *Pelargonium graveolens*

Plant family: Geraniaceae

Type of plant: Plant with shapely leaves and few, small pink flowers

Part used: Leaves and stalks

Method of extraction: Steam distillation

Countries of production: Madagascar (for Bourbon geranium), Egypt, China

When buying, look for: A pale-yellow to light-green watery liquid with a flowery-rose, sweet, soft, green aroma

This is not the ornamental type of geranium known to gardeners. The essential oil is widely used in perfumery. The unique roselike aroma is captured by harvesting the plant just as the leaves turn yellow. Previous to this, the aroma is more lemony. The leaves can be used in cooking.

Caution or Contraindications: None known.

Helichrysum (Italian Everlasting; Immortelle)

Latin name: *Helichrysum italicum*

Plant family: Asteraceae (Compositae)

Type of plant: Bushy herb with very small velvety leaves on long stems, each with a cluster of small yellow flowers

Part used: Flower clusters

Method of extraction: Steam distillation

Countries of production: France (Corsica), Italy, Hungary, Bulgaria

When buying, look for: A pale yellow watery liquid with a powerful, fruity, fresh, strawlike aroma

Listed as a medicinal herb in many Greek, Roman, and medieval European texts. This variety is used for making dry flowers — hence the name Italian everlasting. There are hundreds of helichrysum varieties, but few produce essential oil.

Caution or Contraindications: Avoid during pregnancy or while breastfeeding.

Lavender

Latin name: *Lavandula angustifolia*

Plant family: Labiatae (Lamiaceae)

Type of plant: A bushy herbaceous plant with silver, spike-shaped leaves and flowers in various shades of lavender to purple

Part used: Flowering tops and leaves

Method of extraction: Steam and CO_2 distillation

Countries of production: France, Tasmania, China, England, Bulgaria, Croatia

When buying, look for: A clear, watery liquid with a fresh, herbaceous, almost floral aroma

Many species of lavender are grown. The most highly prized is wild French lavender, grown at high altitude. Spike lavender and "lavendin" are types that cannot be used as substitutes for real lavender, as they have different therapeutic properties. The word *lavender* is derived from the Latin word *lavera*, "to wash," as the ancient Romans used the flowers in their baths.

Caution or Contraindications: None known.

Nutmeg

Latin name: *Myristica fragrans*

Plant family: Myristicaceae

Type of plant: Tall evergreen tree with yellow flowers and large nuts

Part used: Nut

Method of extraction: Steam distillation

Countries of production: Grenada, Sri Lanka, Indonesia

When buying, look for: A watery liquid, yellow to deep orange in color, with a sweet, warm, spicy aroma

Native to the Moluccas Islands, the nutmeg has a long history of use. Wars were fought over access to nutmeg, with the Portuguese trying to keep its source a secret. It was later discovered by the Dutch, and then the British, who introduced the plant to the West Indies — where the best species is now grown. It takes fifteen to twenty years before the tree produces nuts.

Caution or Contraindications: Not to be used during pregnancy. Can cause irritation on sensitive skin — use with care. This is a strong essential oil and should be used with caution. Do not use more than is recommended in blends.

Rose Otto

Latin name: *Rosa damascena*

Plant family: Rosaceae

Type of plant: Bush with large pink flowers

Part used: Fresh flower heads

Method of extraction: Steam distillation

Countries of production: Bulgaria, Turkey, Iran, Cyprus

When buying, look for: A clear liquid with a slight greenish tint and a flowery, rosy, fresh aroma. The liquid can vary between watery and crystalline, depending on whether it's warm or cold, respectively.

In the Kazanlik Valley of Bulgaria, an estimated forty-two square miles of land is taken up by rose production. The roses produce rose oil, rose attar or otto, and rose water. It takes three to four thousand pounds of flowers to make one pound of rose oil, which is why this is one of the most expensive essential oils.

Caution or Contraindications: None known.

CHAPTER TEN

Nutritional Supplements

Vitamins, minerals, and trace minerals provide energy and keep tissues and organs working well on the micro level, the level of the cell. Human beings, like all life-forms, are essentially chemical. Our metabolism is a two-way process in which simple substances are transformed into more complex ones (called anabolism), and then the breaking down of those substances (catabolism) into more simple ones again. This process is the business of life at work, silently maintaining health within cells. Metabolism produces waste by-products, including toxins, which are excreted from the body — if the excretion systems are working properly.

Good health very much depends on a healthy metabolism, which in turn depends upon the supply of nutrients the body requires to carry on its job of building up new cells and disposing of old, unwanted cell material. This is where supplements come in: they make sure we have the building blocks for anabolism and the tools to carry out catabolism.

In an ideal world, there would be no need to take dietary supplements, because our food and drink would provide all the nutrients we need. As it is, modern life is far from ideal. Although we have access to a wide variety of foods from all over the world that should, in principle, provide us with the variety of nutrients we need, many foodstuffs are depleted of their nutritive value. We all know why. Fruit and vegetables are grown using biocides — pesticides, herbicides, and fungicides. In many places the soil itself is often depleted of minerals as a result of monoculture and overfarming and has been treated with nitrates and other chemicals that have, over time, changed its natural structure. Food is frozen or stored for long periods of time, waxed, irradiated, and generally processed; it may look like a piece of fresh raw fruit, vegetable, or herb, but appearances, as they say, can be deceiving.

With so much of what we eat processed in one way or another, our foods are no longer guaranteed to have the expected vitamins. Moreover, they are likely to contain chemical residues that may be harmful to our bodies. We take vitamins and other supplements to replenish the vital building blocks of life and health.

TESTING

There is a large number of available supplements, and the inexperienced may become confused when shopping for them. The first question must be: "What do I need?" Tests can determine whether you are deficient in any vital nutrients, and these are most often available through physicians or qualified nutritionists.

The B vitamins can be tested individually (such as B_1, thiamine; B_2, riboflavin; and B_6, pyridoxine) to see if levels are normal or poor. Tests are also available for other vitamins and the essential fatty acids. There are also standard tests to ascertain levels of minerals and metals, including calcium, magnesium, phosphorus, sodium, potassium, iron, copper, zinc, chromium, manganese, selenium, nickel, cobalt, lead, mercury, cadmium, arsenic, and aluminum. Even lactose intolerance can be deduced, by a breath hydrogen test.

If you do not have access to testing facilities or professional dietary advice, you may wish to take a multivitamin and mineral supplement to ensure that your basic levels of nutrients are maintained so repair and healing can take place. Purchase supplements that are free of yeast, dairy, gluten, and sugar. As the capsules themselves are often made from animal products, it is advisable to purchase those suitable for vegans, which do not utilize these materials.

Vitamins and minerals work as a dynamic integrated system within the body, helping each other to be assimilated and work effectively. If you plan to take an individual vitamin or mineral, take a multivitamin or mineral supplement at the same time to ensure you have at least some of the other nutrients required to metabolize or process it. If you intend to take large amounts over a long period of time, it is best to find out more about how vitamins and minerals work together, to ensure you have a sufficient amount of the supportive supplements required for their safe assimilation.

Nutritional supplementation is a complex subject. Each person has different requirements depending on his or her current dietary intake, lifestyle, and genetics. What might be good for one woman might not be appropriate for another. Also, as there are differing professional suggestions to consider, it would be ideal to get advice from two or more sources concerning the supplements that are best suited to your current situation.

HOW AND WHEN TO TAKE SUPPLEMENTS

Supplements are usually swallowed with water, sprinkled over food, or taken sublingually (absorbed under the tongue). The recommended times for taking them in relation to meals varies, as noted in the table "When to Take Nutritional Supplements."

WHEN TO TAKE NUTRITIONAL SUPPLEMENTS	
TYPE OF SUPPLEMENT	**WHEN TO TAKE IT**
Water-soluble vitamins: B and C	With food or on an empty stomach
Fat-soluble nutrients: Vitamins A, D, and E, essential fatty acids, Co-Q10	With food
(Continued on next page)	

WHEN TO TAKE NUTRITIONAL SUPPLEMENTS (*CONTINUED*)

TYPE OF SUPPLEMENT	WHEN TO TAKE IT
Minerals (except zinc)	With food
Zinc	Before sleeping
Amino acids	2–3 hours before, or after, food
Herbs	Most effective when taken between meals, but can be taken either with food or on an empty stomach

VITAMINS, MINERALS, AND OTHER NUTRIENTS RECOMMENDED FOR WOMEN WITH ENDOMETRIOSIS

What follows is a list of the vitamins and minerals that many nutritional experts feel can be of help to women with endometriosis. These are best obtained from food sources, and these sources are detailed in the chart "Dietary Sources of Vitamins and Minerals" on pages 204–8. However, as many foods are depleted of their nutrients as a result of modern farming, storage, and shipping practices, supplementation may be required. As there is no absolute consensus on the recommended daily intake, and because this depends upon the diet of the individual woman, it may be wise at the outset to simply follow the manufacturer's instructions.

Vitamins

From a consumer's point of view, there are two types of vitamin: water soluble and fat soluble. The water-soluble vitamins — such as B and C — cannot be stored in the body and are excreted within a day. This is why they have to be taken regularly, usually once a day. Fat-soluble vitamins, such as A, D, E, and K, can be taken less often because they are stored in the liver and in fatty tissue.

Another important distinction in vitamin supplements is that some are natural and some are synthetic. Natural vitamins are derived from fruit and other food sources, while synthetic vitamins are put together chemically following the blueprint of the natural molecule. In nature, however, nutrient elements are linked together in a complex way not yet entirely understood; the synthetic copies are simpler and may be less effective. Synthetic copies also tend to have additives such as coloring, sugar, and starch, and surprises like coal tar.

The commercial manufacture of vitamins involves the use of excipients, compounds that hold the ingredients together, or add bulk to the capsule, or allow the product to be free-flowing for production, or serve as a coating agent. Excipients should be natural as well. Among those commonly used in natural vitamin production are lecithin, vegetable oil, acacia gum, alfa alfa, stearic acid, microcrystalline cellulose, and hypomellose — all derived from plant material.

Vitamin A

Women whose menstrual flow is excessive have lower levels of vitamin A. Aside from limiting the amount of menstrual bleeding, vitamin A is vital to the nervous system, boosts immunity, and is necessary for the repair of epithelial tissue, such as the mucous membrane. However, too much vitamin A can be toxic. This vitamin should not be taken during pregnancy unless under medical advice. As it's thought that too much might affect the activity of genes, it may be wise to obtain medical advice before taking vitamin A.

Beta-carotene, which comes from plants, is a precursor of vitamin A and is vital to vitamin A production. It is water soluble, as opposed to vitamin A, which is fat soluble.

B Vitamins

B vitamins are water soluble and must be taken daily because they are excreted within a day. This is a large group of essential nutrients, including:

- B_1: thiamine
- B_2: riboflavin
- B_3: niacin (also called nicotinic acid)
- B_5: pantothenic acid
- B_6: pyridoxine
- B_{12}: cyanocobalamin
- Other elements, such as biotin and choline, which are grouped with the B vitamins

Each B vitamin has unique properties. They are not related chemically, which may come as a surprise, but their functions are interrelated and they work synergistically with each other as a group. If you find you are lacking in one B vitamin, it's quite possible you are lacking in others in the B group.

Women who fall into the following categories are often deficient in B vitamins: those who take oral contraceptives or cortisone or have recently taken antibiotics; those who eat a lot of refined sugar or are alcoholic or experience PMS. The B vitamins may play a part in regulating the menstrual cycle, for two reasons: they help reduce stress, which affects the cycle; and they contribute to good adrenal and thyroid hormone production. In addition, B vitamins aid in the production of the "good" prostaglandins, which are anti-inflammatory and help relax the uterine muscle.

Symptoms of B Vitamin Deficiency May Include:

- Menstrual cramps or pain
- Irregular periods
- Premenstrual syndrome
- Fluid retention
- Depression
- Anxiety
- Moodiness
- Stress
- Lack of concentration
- Fatigue or lack of energy
- Weight problems
- Bad breath
- Headaches
- Eczema
- Dandruff
- Sensitivity to light
- Cracked and sore lips and mouth corners
- Tongue enlarged or decreased in size, or smooth and sore

Benefits of B Vitamins

- Regulate liver function and help the liver break down excess estrogen
- Help metabolize fats and proteins
- Provide components of enzymes that generate new cells
- Assist the body in forming energy from foods
- Help maintain healthy skin
- Aid in proper function of brain and nervous system
- Assist in the production of red blood cells
- Assist in breaking down carbohydrates
- Help maintain healthy intestinal muscle
- Help maintain healthy eyes

Vitamin B_1: Thiamine. Thiamine levels tend to be depleted in the body if a woman has been taking oral contraceptives or antibiotics, or if she consumes a great deal of caffeine or alcohol. The tannin in tea can act against B_1.

Symptoms of Vitamin B_1 (Thiamine) Deficiency May Include:

- Gastrointestinal disturbances
- Constipation
- Loss of appetite
- Severe weight loss
- Enlarged liver
- Water retention (edema)
- Sore, weak, or atrophied muscles
- Tingling and numbness of the hands and feet
- Fatigue
- Forgetfulness
- Irritability
- Nervousness

Benefits of Vitamin B_1

- Acts as an antioxidant
- Metabolizes carbohydrates
- Assists in blood formation
- Stimulates circulation
- Restores muscle tone of the heart, intestines, and stomach
- Stimulates energy
- Restores normal appetite and growth
- Improves learning capacity

Vitamin B$_2$: Riboflavin. Riboflavin levels tend to be depleted if a woman has been taking oral contraceptives or antibiotics, doing strenuous exercise, or drinking large quantities of alcohol. It's important to follow the recommended daily allowance, because cataracts and other eye problems can be caused by overconsumption of this vitamin. B$_2$ is one of the vitamins recommended during pregnancy.

Symptoms of Vitamin B$_2$ (Riboflavin) Deficiency May Include:

- Poor digestion
- Inflammation of mouth and tongue
- Insomnia
- Dizziness
- Light sensitivity
- Eye disorders
- Cracks and sores at corner of mouth
- Dermatitis
- Hair loss

Benefits of Vitamin B$_2$

- Metabolizes carbohydrates, fats, and proteins
- Assists in red blood cell formation
- Assists in antibody formation
- Assists in cell growth
- Assists in cell respiration
- Prevents and treats cataracts
- Prevents eye fatigue
- Aids in the absorption of iron and vitamin B$_6$

Vitamin B$_3$: Niacin. There are two forms of this vitamin: niacin (also called nicotinic acid) and niacinamide.

Contraindications
- Do not take B$_3$ (niacin/nicotinic acid or niacinamide) if you

are pregnant, or if you have gout, liver disease, peptic ulcers, or glaucoma.

- Because B_3 may elevate blood sugar levels, seek advice before taking it if you have diabetes.

Symptoms of Vitamin B_3 (Niacin) Deficiency May Include:

- Low blood sugar
- Indigestion
- Diarrhea
- Loss of appetite
- Halitosis
- Muscular weakness
- Limb pains
- Inflammation
- Headaches
- Fatigue
- Dizziness
- Insomnia
- Depression
- Skin eruptions

Benefits of Vitamin B_3

- Helps synthesize hormones
- Aids in the secretion of bile and stomach fluids
- Metabolizes carbohydrates, fats, and proteins
- Stimulates circulation
- Lowers cholesterol
- Aids in the function of the nervous system

Vitamin B_5: Pantothenic Acid. Vitamin B_5 is crucial for the production of adrenal gland hormones, including small amounts of estrogen, progesterone, and testosterone. The adrenals also regulate the metabolism of proteins, fats, and carbohydrates, which is why, perhaps, B_5 can give such an effective energy boost. B_5 is often referred to as the antistress hormone and has also been found to help in cases of anxiety and depression. B_5 is linked to ovarian hormone activity and neurotransmitter production — brain chemical activity.

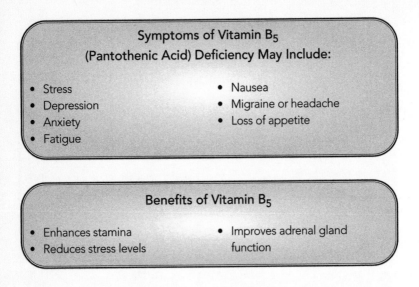

Symptoms of Vitamin B$_5$
(Pantothenic Acid) Deficiency May Include:

- Stress
- Depression
- Anxiety
- Fatigue

- Nausea
- Migraine or headache
- Loss of appetite

Benefits of Vitamin B$_5$

- Enhances stamina
- Reduces stress levels

- Improves adrenal gland function

Vitamin B6: Pyridoxine. B6 is an especially useful vitamin as it is involved in a wide range of body functions. It may become depleted in women who are taking oral contraceptives, estrogen therapy, diuretics, cortisone drugs, or antidepressants. To get the most B6 from food, steam or boil vegetables for as short a time as possible, in very little water, and roast or grill meats.

Contraindications
- There has been some suggestion that high doses (300 milligrams a day) used over long periods of time may be toxic.

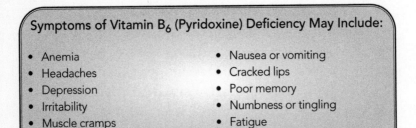

Symptoms of Vitamin B$_6$ (Pyridoxine) Deficiency May Include:

- Anemia
- Headaches
- Depression
- Irritability
- Muscle cramps
- Acne or oily skin

- Nausea or vomiting
- Cracked lips
- Poor memory
- Numbness or tingling
- Fatigue

Benefits of Vitamin B$_6$

- Reduces menstrual pain or cramps
- Aids in "good" prostaglandin production
- Helps rid body of excess estrogen
- Balances hormones
- Aids in red blood cell production
- Helps maintain the sodium-potassium balance
- Aids liver function
- Essential for nervous system
- Essential for brain function
- Aids in the synthesis of DNA and RNA
- Assists in the absorption of fats and proteins
- Aids in the production of certain enzymes
- Acts as a diuretic

B$_{12}$: Cyanocobalamin. Vitamin B$_{12}$ is needed by every cell in the body because it's required for the synthesis of DNA. Without it, there can be problems not only with cell formation and preservation but also in the synthesis of proteins and in the body's ability to absorb food and utilize it correctly. B$_{12}$ is also vital to the nervous system, because it helps maintain the fatty sheaths that surround nerve endings.

B$_{12}$ in the body can be destroyed by large quantities of vitamin C taken over a prolonged period of time. The absorption of vitamin B$_{12}$ can also be blocked by overuse of potassium supplements and certain anticoagulant drugs.

Symptoms of Vitamin B$_{12}$ (Cyanocobalamin) Deficiency May Include:

- Anemia
- Heart palpitations
- Fatigue
- Headaches or migraines
- Dizzy spells
- Nervous disorders, including irritability, moodiness, and depression
- Liver enlargement

> ## Benefits of Vitamin B$_{12}$
>
> - Helps in the uptake of iron
> - Aids sleep
> - Improves fertility
> - Helps metabolize fats and carbohydrates

Biotin. A good supply of biotin is required for the efficient working of many basic body mechanisms, including the production of bone marrow and cells. Biotin is manufactured in the intestines and is vital to fatty acid production and the absorption of other B vitamins. Antibiotics and saccharin can reduce the body's ability to produce biotin from foods.

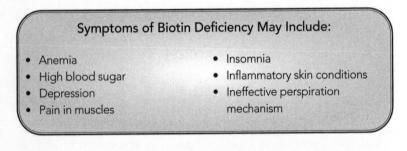

> ## Symptoms of Biotin Deficiency May Include:
>
> - Anemia
> - High blood sugar
> - Depression
> - Pain in muscles
> - Insomnia
> - Inflammatory skin conditions
> - Ineffective perspiration mechanism

> ## Benefits of Biotin
>
> - Helps maintain a healthy nervous system
> - Relieves muscular pain

Choline. Choline is required for a wide range of body functions, especially those relating to the liver, kidneys, heart, and fertility. Since choline is required for processing fats, a deficiency can cause a buildup of fat in the liver. The gallbladder can also be affected. Because choline is involved in lecithin production, a deficiency can cause problems in the nervous system.

Symptoms of Choline Deficiency May Include:

- Fatty degeneration or cirrhosis of the liver
- Raised cholesterol
- Gastric ulcers
- Kidney problems
- Hardening of the arteries
- Poor memory

Benefits of Choline

- Aids in hormone production
- Enhances fertility
- Aids in liver function
- Improves nerve impulse transmission
- Regulates gallbladder

Folic Acid (or Folate). Folic acid is required for cell division and DNA replication. Red and white blood cells cannot form or function well without it. The most usual cause of deficiency is a lack of fresh fruit and vegetables, although overcooking vegetables also destroys what folic acid is present. Folic acid is especially needed by women taking oral contraceptives, and it is best combined with vitamins B_{12} and C.

Contraindications
- Consult your physician before taking folic acid if you have cancer or epilepsy.

Symptoms of Folic Acid Deficiency May Include:

- Sore or red tongue
- Anemia
- General weakness or disinterest in life
- Tiredness
- Insomnia
- Bad memory

Benefits of Folic Acid

- Aids in healthy cell formation
- Improves immune system
- Improves energy levels
- Improves sleep

Vitamin C

Human beings do not have the enzyme needed to produce vitamin C. A very small amount can be converted from folic acid, but, as that is also sometimes deficient, production of vitamin C is often extremely low. Vitamin C has to be obtained from food. We require at least five servings of fruit and vegetables a day. If we do not take in enough vitamin C this way, supplementation is required.

The most effective form of vitamin C is known as "esterified." It is absorbed into the body far more quickly than the standard form because it contains vitamin C metabolites that are the same as those our bodies make. Vitamin C supplements are best when combined with bioflavonoids (see below), and the daily dose should be halved and taken on two occasions during the day. Vitamin C is said to play a part in over three hundred metabolic processes, making it one of the most important vitamins to have in plentiful supply. The doses recommended often seem very high, and if you experience diarrhea, this generally indicates bowel intolerance and you may be taking too much.

Vitamin C is important to women with endometriosis because it strengthens the tiny veins, the capillaries, and may help reduce menstrual bleeding. Vitamin C works in all kinds of ways to benefit the body. It is needed for the metabolism of nutrients, increases the absorption of vital elements such as iron, and is required for the production of certain proteins, including interferon, which blocks the synthesis of viral proteins, and so reduces infection.

The lymphocytes that fight infection replicate using a type of cell division known as phytohemagglutinin-induced blastogenesis. The flu virus works by preventing this process, and vitamin C switches it on again. This is where the battle in the body takes place — and you need vitamin C to fight the fight. Vitamin C also boosts prostaglandin E production in blood platelets, increasing lymphocyte production.

As well as making us feel better by improving the immune system, vitamin C helps us look better by helping form the collagen that supports the skin, and it helps us live longer by protecting against blood clotting. Vitamin C helps heal wounds, including burns, and aids the function of the adrenal glands. Vitamin C is also an antioxidant and plays an important part in detoxification. Not only does it help detoxify the harmful by-products of many bacteria, but it can also latch on to heavy metals in the body, making them inactive and more easily eliminated from the body.

Vitamin C is particularly needed by women who drink a lot of alcohol, smoke, or regularly take aspirin or other painkillers, oral contraceptives, steroids, antidepressants, and other medical drugs. Women who are diabetic often need vitamin C, but, as it can affect the uptake of diabetes medications, they must consult their physicians before taking supplements. Vitamin C can also reduce the symptoms of asthma, but women with this condition should consult their physicians first concerning the dosages they can take.

Contraindications
- If pregnant, consult your physician about the amount of vitamin C you can safely take at this time.
- Women with diabetes should consult their physicians before taking supplements.
- Irritation of the stomach can occur if standard vitamin C (ascorbic acid) is taken at the same time as aspirin, possibly leading to ulcers.
- Tooth enamel may be damaged by the chewable form of vitamin C.

> ## Symptoms of Vitamin C Deficiency May Include:
>
> - Frequent infections
> - Easy bruising
> - Bleeding gums or bad teeth
> - Joint pain
> - Fatigue
> - Digestive problems

> ## Benefits of Vitamin C
>
> - Strengthens immune system
> - Has antiviral properties
> - Strengthens bones and joints
> - Improves condition of skin
> - Gives mild pain relief

Bioflavonoids

Bioflavonoids are mostly found in fruit — particularly citrus fruit — and in some vegetables. In foods they are found in conjunction with vitamin C, and they are thought to improve the action of vitamin C, either by enhancing the body's ability to absorb it, or by protecting vitamin C from being oxidized.

There are many different bioflavonoids, including hesperidin and rutin, both of which have been referred to as vitamin P. The human body cannot produce bioflavonoids, and so these must be supplied in the form of fruit or a supplement.

Bioflavonoids contribute to strengthening the capillary walls and so encourage good circulation while also reducing bleeding. Spider veins, bruising, and varicose veins may indicate bioflavonoid deficiency. They help reduce inflammation by deactivating the enzymes that cause inflammation. Quercetin is one of the bioflavonoids thought to reduce inflammation, and it also inhibits the release of histamine, which helps allergy sufferers. Bioflavonoids are said to relax smooth muscles, prevent inflammation, relieve pain, and act as a mild antibacterial agent.

Vitamin E

Vitamin E is a term applied to eight different molecules, of which alpha-tocopherol is the strongest and most recommended form. Vitamin E is well known as an antioxidant and is widely used for skin repair, both medically and cosmetically. Its youth-giving effects on the exterior, the skin, are mirrored on the interior of the body. In particular, vitamin E helps maintain the integrity of the cell membranes, capillary walls, red blood cells, nerves, and muscles. Vitamin E helps protect the body from the effects of pollution and may be particularly valuable to women living in urban environments.

Contraindications

• If you have a heart condition or are taking anticoagulant medication, consult your physician before taking this supplement.

• Care should also be taken if you have diabetes or an overactive thyroid gland.

Symptoms of Vitamin E Deficiency May Include:

• Premenstrual syndrome
• Heavy menstrual bleeding
• Infertility
• Easy bruising
• Loss of muscle tone
• Leg cramps

Benefits of Vitamin E

• Helps to balance hormones
• Improves fertility
• Improves circulation
• Improves healing
• Reduces scarring

Vitamin K

Although vitamin K can be obtained from some food and herb sources, most is synthesized in the intestines by "friendly" bacteria. When antibiotics are taken, they often destroy not only the "bad" but also the "good" bacteria, and vitamin K production is disturbed. For this reason, women who have been on antibiotics for long periods of time should consider whether they need vitamin K supplementation.

Vitamin K converts glucose into glycogen, which is required for a healthy liver. It also produces prothrombin, which is required for blood clotting. A deficiency of vitamin K may be partly responsible in some cases of abnormal bleeding.

Essential Fatty Acids

Every cell in the body needs essential fatty acids (EFAs), which can be seen as the fat element of life's building blocks. The body doesn't produce them, so EFAs must be included in the diet. If they are not, supplementation is recommended. Evening primrose oil is widely used in cases of premenstrual syndrome and is perhaps the best-known EFA, but many other useful EFAs can be added to the diet. It is said that EFAs should represent 10–20 percent of daily calorie intake, but it is often difficult to ingest this amount given modern eating patterns.

For women with endometriosis, EFAs are important for several reasons. They are precursors to prostaglandins, which are a form of hormone or chemical messenger. There are "good" and "bad" prostaglandins, and it's the bad form that is thought to account for much of the inflammation and pain of endometriosis. If the EFAs are not present in the diet, an imbalance, with an excess of the "bad" prostaglandins, may develop. Make sure you have enough vitamin B6, zinc, and magnesium, because these help metabolize EFAs into the "good" prostaglandins (PGE1 and PGE3). For the body to function, it must be well oxygenated, and EFAs increase our ability to metabolize oxygen, making it available for the body to use. EFAs also increase our overall metabolic rate and, in this way, contribute to weight loss. Because excess estrogen is stored in body fat, a loss of weight can mean a loss of excess estrogen and a reduction of the symptoms of endometriosis.

Essential fatty acids are crucial to the cardiovascular system because they lower triglycerides — fats — in the blood, as well as in the tissue. This helps keep the arteries clear and arteriosclerosis at bay. Omega-6 also helps prevent blockage of the arteries and blood clotting while at the same time preventing the constriction of blood vessels.

There are water-soluble and fat-soluble elements in the body and, just as vitamin C is an antioxidant for the water-based elements of our body, EFAs play the antioxidant role in the fat-based elements. The brain is the most fat-concentrated part of the human body, and EFAs account for half its weight. It should come as no surprise, then, to learn that a lack of EFAs can have a detrimental effect on learning and behavior — particularly noticeable in children. A lack of EFAs has also been shown to contribute to depression in adults.

Contraindications
• Do not take fish oil supplements if you have diabetes; consume fresh fish instead.

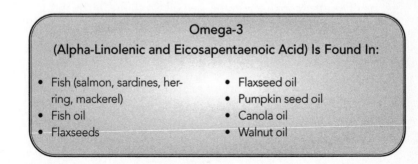

Omega-3
(Alpha-Linolenic and Eicosapentaenoic Acid) Is Found In:

- Fish (salmon, sardines, herring, mackerel)
- Fish oil
- Flaxseeds
- Flaxseed oil
- Pumpkin seed oil
- Canola oil
- Walnut oil

Omega-6 (Linoleic Acid and Gamma-Linolenic Acid, or GLA) Is Found In:

- Evening primrose oil
- Safflower oil
- Sunflower oil
- Walnut oil
- Sesame oil
- Pumpkin seed oil
- Pistachio nut oil
- Borage (starflower) oil
- Almond oil
- Grape seed oil
- Canola oil
- Seeds
- Nuts

Omega-9 (Oleic Acid) Is Found In:

- Olive oil
- Hazelnut oil
- Almond oil
- Canola oil
- Pistachio oil
- Sesame oil
- Pumpkin seed oil
- Walnut oil
- Sunflower oil
- Flaxseed oil
- Safflower oil

The quality of the oil determines the amount of EFAs. It is important to purchase organically grown and "cold-pressed" oils packaged in opaque containers. They should be stored away from heat and light, as these can destroy the EFAs. The only oil that is said to retain its EFAs after cooking is grape seed oil, so all the others must be used raw — uncooked. They can be mixed in salad dressings, drizzled over pasta, rice, or vegetables, and even stirred into oatmeal or added to drinks.

As with so much that is health related, making small informed changes in dietary habits may have a tremendous effect on the body. EFAs are better for your health than many of the overprocessed oils more routinely consumed. The production of margarine, for example, converts the very good linoleic acid into trans-fatty acids, which should be avoided by women with endometriosis.

Probiotics

There are around five hundred species of bacteria in the healthy human gastrointestinal (GI) system. Some are known to be benign or harmless, and others are harmful. Most of the time, the bacteria and other microorganisms inside our guts live out their lives without causing us any harm and, in fact, perform many physical services we need for a healthy life. Sometimes, though, the "friendly" bacteria get depleted, allowing the "bad" bacteria to reproduce unopposed and run out of control, causing physical problems. This might happen as a result of something specific, such as taking a course of antibiotics or having food poisoning, or it may be caused by a chronic condition, such as irritable bowel syndrome. Nutritional deficiency or chronic stress may also be at the root of the problem.

Symptoms of GI Flora Imbalance May Include:

- Overgrowth of *Candida albicans*
- Poor immune system
- Allergies
- Constipation

Benefits of GI Flora Balance

- Improves digestion of proteins
- Helps maintain a healthy elimination system
- Improves absorption of nutrients
- Improves immune system

The aim of probiotics is to introduce more "good" bacteria into the gastrointestinal tract: the stomach, duodenum, jejunum, ileum, and large intestine. Different bacteria colonize these different areas according to, in part, the amount of oxygen they need. Lactobacillus species live higher in the tract, where there is more oxygen, and bifidobacteria tend to concentrate lower in the tract, where there is less oxygen. As these two species restore balance to the intestinal "flora," probiotic therapy largely consists of ingesting these organisms. Probably the best known of the "friendly" bacteria is lactobicillus acidophilus; dairy-free forms are available.

For a woman with endometriosis, it is important that excess estrogens be excreted from the body. The final stage of this process is sometimes disturbed by the activity of a bacterial enzyme, beta-glucuronidase, which detaches estrogens from bile so they are reabsorbed into the body instead of excreted in fecal matter. To prevent this, take probiotics or the supplement calcium D-glucarate (200–300 milligrams a day), which will help control beta-glucuronidase activity. Calcium D-glucarate occurs naturally in certain fruits and vegetables, including apples, grapefruit, broccoli, and other cruciferous vegetables. Also helpful is a reduction in your intake of animal fat, which encourages the growth of bacteria that produce the unhelpful beta-glucuronidase.

Minerals

Although only a tiny percentage of the human body is composed of minerals — including iron, zinc, calcium, magnesium, and potassium — they are vital to the healthy functioning of the body.

Iron

Iron deficiency is quite common in women who are menstruating or have rheumatoid arthritis, and in some vegetarians. Women with candidiasis, heavy menstrual bleeding, or chronic herpes infections also often show a deficiency.

A deficiency most usually develops through insufficient intake of foods rich in iron, but it can also be brought about by too much tea or coffee or a diet high in phosphorus. Anemia is sometimes caused by a deficiency in vitamins B_6 or B_{12}. Poor digestion, use of antacids, ulcers, and long-term illness can deplete iron stores.

Another rare, but important, cause of iron deficiency is internal bleeding. Any suspicion of this should be referred to your physician.

The correct dose to take is difficult to judge, and professional advice may be required. According to some experts, only 10 percent of iron supplementation is absorbed. This may partly result from insufficient hydrochloric acid in the stomach. Or it may be because there is insufficient copper, manganese, molybdenum, or vitamin A or B complex, or because there is an excess of vitamin E or zinc. Too much iron can also increase the need for vitamin E. Vitamin C is said to increase iron absorption by 30 percent. On the other hand, heavy exercise and perspiration can deplete iron.

With all these different things to consider, you can see that it's important to have a wide profile of your present vitamin and mineral status before embarking on a program of supplementation.

Although a certain amount of iron is required to keep the immune system working well, too much iron can have the reverse effect and suppress the immune system while also leading to the production of more free radicals. For this reason, iron should be taken with a degree of caution.

Contraindications
- It may not be wise to take iron supplements while you have a bacterial infection, as bacteria need iron to grow.
- Overuse of iron supplementation can lead to constipation.

Symptoms of Iron Deficiency May Include:

- Anemia
- Brittle hair
- Lengthwise ridges on nails
- Fragile bones
- Fatigue
- Nervousness
- Inflammation in mouth
- Difficulty swallowing
- Digestive problems

Benefits of Iron

- Improves antibody production, leading to better immune response
- Oxygenates red blood cells
- Improves production of enzymes involved in energy production
- Strengthens muscle tissue

Zinc

Zinc is found in over two hundred of the body's enzymes, including superoxide dismutase, which is an antioxidant. Free radical production is prevented by zinc. It also contributes to protein synthesis and fatty acid metabolism, and is a component of insulin. The immune system is strengthened by zinc, partly because T cells are matured with the hormone thymulin, the production of which requires zinc. The liver is protected from chemical damage by zinc. As if all this were not enough, zinc also contributes to cell replication, which makes it crucial to every element of our lives. Yet the total amount of zinc in a 140-pound body is just 2.10 grams.

As with all the vitamins and minerals, there are complex interactions. Zinc is particularly required to maintain vitamins A and E in the body. Zinc should be taken with calcium and magnesium, but not with iron because they seem to counteract each other's activity. Zinc is only absorbed at night, so take it before going to bed. Zinc gluconate is most often recommended as having the best rate of absorption. Nutritionists tell us that copper and zinc should be maintained at the correct ratio, but they fail to agree on what that is. And finding where to get tested for mineral levels is not easy.

Zinc deficiency can occur in areas where there are still copper water pipes, and even hard water can be responsible. Depletion can result from eating an overabundance of fiber or legumes because they contain phytates that bind with zinc, so it's excreted rather than absorbed by the body. Zinc can also be lost through diarrhea and, it is said, excessive perspiration. Zinc levels can be lowered by diabetes, cirrhosis of the liver, or kidney disease.

Contraindications
• It has been suggested by some medical professionals that it is inadvisable to take zinc supplements if you have cancer, as zinc is required for cell replication.

Symptoms of Zinc Deficiency May Include:

• Infertility
• Inability to taste or smell
• White spots on nails
• Thin or peeling nails
• Depression
• Headaches
• Irritability
• Acne
• Fatigue
• High cholesterol levels

Benefits of Zinc

• Reduces menstrual cramps
• Improves immune function
• Aids in antioxidant activity
• Assists insulin activity
• Creates strong bones
• Improves tissue repair
• Improves skin, hair, and nails

Selenium
Selenium illustrates some of the difficulties that arise when considering taking supplements. While it is certainly a vital trace element, having too much in the body can cause almost as many problems as having too little. It is difficult to ensure an adequate supply, though, because selenium levels in the soil can be very low, as they are in much of the United States, Britain, and New Zealand. For this reason, it may actually be helpful to consume foods from different countries, rather than relying entirely on local produce.

The ultimate difficulty, of course, is that few people know their selenium level and, as its content in food is uncertain, it is almost impossible to know how to improve it. While a deficiency in selenium has been linked to cancer and heart disease, too-high selenium levels have been linked to arthritis and kidney impairment. Too-high selenium levels might be indicated by a metallic taste in the mouth, yellowish skin, or brittle nails, among other symptoms.

Selenium is present in a wide range of foods and herbs, including meats and grains. But how much is present depends on the source. While the animals grazing on New Zealand soil can become depleted of selenium, New Zealanders who eat them are not particularly deficient in selenium because they import a lot of Australian wheat — which does contain selenium. You can see how complex the subject of nutritional supplements has become.

It is also difficult to find agreement among nutritionists as to the correct amount to take — recommendations vary from 50 micrograms per day to 200. Its always better to take less than more unless you are under medical supervision. Another factor to consider is that selenium works together with vitamin E, which is why nutritionists often recommend taking them both at the same time.

Selenium is a good antioxidant, especially when working with vitamin E. In particular it prevents oxidation of lipids, or fats, in the body. It also prevents the production of free radicals and helps in the production of antibodies, which benefits the immune system.

Contraindications
•   Assess your levels of selenium before embarking on a course
    of supplementation. Instead, take a multivitamin that in-
    cludes selenium.

Symptoms of Selenium Deficiency May Include:

- Menstrual cramps
- Infections
- High cholesterol
- Tiredness

> ### Benefits of Selenium
>
> - Improves pancreas function
> - Improves liver function
> - Improves the immune system
> - Contributes to a healthy heart
> - Increases tissue elasticity

Calcium

Estrogen helps deposit calcium in the bones, which is why, after menopause, when estrogen production is reduced, our bones can develop osteoporosis. Ninety-nine percent of the calcium in our bodies can be found in the bones; the remaining 1 percent is found in blood and other body fluids and in soft tissue. Although 1 percent might not sound significant, this small amount of calcium is vital to many body functions. Of particular interest to us is the fact that a calcium deficiency can affect muscle tone and contribute to menstrual cramping. Because calcium levels begin to drop about ten days before menstruation begins, and are lowest just before menstruation, low calcium levels might be a contributing factor in premenstrual syndrome.

Calcium absorption can be disturbed by heavy exercise regimes and by quite a few dietary factors. Foods containing certain acids inhibit the absorption of calcium, including chocolate, rhubarb, and spinach. Grains and fizzy drinks that are high in phosphorus encourage the excretion of calcium, as do coffee, alcohol, and packaged foods high in salt. In general, diets high in fats, protein, or sugar prevent calcium utilization, and foods containing the amino acid lysine encourage calcium absorption. These helpful foods include lean red meat, fish, dairy products, eggs, soy, lima beans, potatoes, and yeast. Calcium absorption is also disturbed by a lack of sunshine — which produces vitamin D in us — and the presence in the body of heavy metals such as lead and aluminum.

It is important to maintain calcium at normal levels, because calcium is crucial to the body's proper functioning. On the cellular level, calcium contributes to the formation of RNA and DNA, helps keep the cell membranes permeable, and maintains healthy neuro-muscular activity and blood clotting. Calcium is involved in the man-ufacture of enzymes necessary for a range of activities, from immune system function to the breakdown of fats.

There are many different types of calcium supplements. Cal-cium citrate is easily absorbed. In general, citrates, ascorbates, and chelated types are recommended, while carbons, oxides, sulfates, and chlorides are not. D1-calcium-phosphate is insoluble, and it may disturb the body's ability to absorb a multivitamin and mineral sup-plement.

Contraindications
- Do not take calcium supplementation if you have kidney stones.
- If on medication for heart problems, seek advice from your physician before taking calcium supplements.

Symptoms of Calcium Deficiency May Include:

- Muscle cramps
- Numbness in limbs
- Tooth decay or inflamed gums
- Depression or hyperactivity
- Rheumatoid arthritis
- Heart palpitations
- Brittle nails
- Eczema

Benefits of Calcium

- Reduces menstrual cramps
- Enhances sleep
- Lowers cholesterol
- Lowers blood pressure
- Improves energy levels
- Improves skin tone

Magnesium

Magnesium is an extremely important nutrient because a deficiency can play a part in cardiac arrest. Magnesium is particularly important for a woman with endometriosis, because it helps convert essential fatty acids to "good" prostaglandins, as opposed to "bad" prostaglandins — which are thought to be the cause of much of the pain associated with endometriosis. Magnesium is also a muscle relaxant and has been shown in research to reduce menstrual pain.

As magnesium has an effect on the neuromuscular system, a deficiency can have wide-ranging results, from nervousness and depression to muscle weakness and twitching. Magnesium contributes to the formation of bones and reduces the risk of osteoporosis. It is important for the metabolism of potassium, and, along with vitamin D, for the efficient absorption of calcium. Taken along with B6, it may help dissolve calcium phosphate, or "kidney stones." Magnesium is also said to prevent calcification of soft tissue and reduce cholesterol, as well as strengthen the lining of the arteries and prevent cardiovascular disease. It is a vital catalyst in enzyme activity, and it encourages carbohydrate metabolism and the conversion of linoleic acid to gamma-linoleic acid. Magnesium also helps maintain the proper pH balance in the body.

A depletion of magnesium can be caused by diarrhea; the long-term use of diuretics or fat-soluble vitamins; the overconsumption of alcohol, tea, almonds, spinach, rhubarb, cocoa, or cod-liver oil; or a diet rich in protein or fats. High levels of vitamin D or zinc can interfere with magnesium uptake, as can calcium. Magnesium should be taken in a 1:2 proportion with calcium (1 magnesium to 2 calcium; 250 milligrams magnesium to 500 milligrams calcium gluconate). There are different types of magnesium, including taurate, which is said to be good for the breakdown of estrogen, and magnesium malate, which is recommended for fatigue.

Symptoms of Magnesium Deficiency May Include:

- Nervousness or depression
- Chronic pain
- Chronic fatigue
- Dizziness or confusion
- Insomnia
- Irritable bowel syndrome
- Digestive problems
- Premenstrual syndrome

Benefits of Magnesium

- Creates a relaxing effect or reduces stress levels
- Reduces menstrual cramps
- Reduces lower back pain
- Regulates body temperature
- Builds strong bones
- Builds good muscle tone

Potassium

Potassium is a mineral and works in conjunction with sodium, which is a mineral salt. They are both electrolytes and are involved in the transmission of electrochemical impulses. When we are under stress, the body produces certain hormones that deplete the level of potassium in the body and disrupt the potassium-sodium ratio, both outside the cell and within it. Potassium is essential to the process of passing nutrients through the cell membranes, and it is also necessary for chemical reactions to take place within the cells.

Potassium is required for many basic functions, including muscle contraction, nerve transmission, and the ability of the body to maintain good fluid balance. A deficiency can cause salt retention. Potassium is also involved in synthesizing protein from amino acids. A deficiency can affect many body functions, from cognitive ability, mental state — such as nervousness or depression — and glucose intolerance, to digestion, breathing, and sleep. Caffeine, tobacco, diarrhea, and diuretics can reduce the ability of the body to absorb potassium.

Contraindications

- If you have a disorder of the heart or kidneys or are on any medication, medical advice must be sought before taking potassium supplementation.

Symptoms of Potassium Deficiency May Include:

- Excessive thirst
- Muscular fatigue
- Weakness or fatigue
- Diarrhea or constipation
- Acne or dry skin
- Bloating or water retention

Benefits of Potassium

- Reduces menstrual cramps
- Strengthens muscles
- Reduces cholesterol levels
- Improves carbohydrate metabolism

DIETARY SOURCES OF VITAMINS AND MINERALS

FOOD SOURCES	Vit. A	Vit. B	Vit. B1	Vit. B2	Vit. B3	Vit. B5	Vit. B6	Vit. B12	Biotin	Choline	Folic Acid	Vit. C	Bioflavonoids	Vit. E	Vit. K	Iron	Zinc	Calcium	Magnesium	Potassium
Meat (general)	✓				✓	✓	✓	✓	✓	✓							✓		✓	✓
Beef			✓	✓	✓	✓	✓	✓			✓					✓	✓			
Lamb			✓		✓	✓	✓	✓			✓					✓	✓		✓	
Pork			✓	✓	✓	✓	✓	✓			✓					✓	✓		✓	✓
Chicken			✓	✓	✓		✓	✓	✓							✓	✓		✓	✓
Turkey		✓	✓	✓	✓		✓	✓	✓							✓	✓			
Veal		✓	✓	✓	✓	✓	✓	✓									✓			
Liver	✓		✓		✓	✓	✓	✓	✓		✓			✓	✓	✓				
Kidney				✓	✓	✓	✓	✓			✓					✓	✓			
Fish (general)			✓		✓	✓	✓			✓										
Saltwater fish						✓			✓											
Cod																			✓	✓
Flounder																			✓	
Tuna				✓			✓	✓			✓			✓		✓	✓			
Mackerel							✓							✓			✓			
Haddock																	✓			
Herring			✓					✓									✓			
Salmon			✓	✓			✓	✓			✓			✓		✓		✓	✓	✓
Sardine								✓								✓	✓	✓	✓	✓
Shellfish (general)																				
Clam								✓												
Crab								✓												
Lobster						✓													✓	
Oyster				✓												✓	✓			
Shrimp																	✓			
Eggs (general)			✓	✓	✓	✓	✓	✓	✓	✓	✓					✓			✓	
Egg yolks			✓	✓	✓		✓	✓	✓	✓				✓	✓	✓	✓			
Milk (cow's)	✓			✓			✓											✓	✓	✓
Buttermilk																		✓		
Goat's milk																		✓		
Whey																		✓		
Yogurt				✓				✓										✓		
Cheese (general)				✓			✓				✓							✓		
Blue cheese							✓													

FOOD SOURCES	Vit. A	Vit. B	Vit. B₁	Vit. B₂	Vit. B₃	Vit. B₅	Vit. B₆	Vit. B₁₂	Biotin	Choline	Folic Acid	Vit. C	Bioflavonoids	Vit. E	Vit. K	Iron	Zinc	Calcium	Magnesium	Potassium
Cheddar cheese																		✓	✓	
Cottage cheese																✓		✓		
Swiss cheese																		✓		
Vegetables (general)						✓														
Artichokes																				✓
Asparagus	✓	✓	✓	✓							✓				✓	✓		✓		
Aubergine/ Eggplant																			✓	
Avocados	✓		✓	✓		✓	✓					✓				✓			✓	✓
Beans: green	✓		✓	✓		✓				✓				✓			✓		✓	
Kidney beans			✓	✓			✓				✓					✓			✓	
Lima beans		✓														✓			✓	✓
Soybeans		✓	✓		✓			✓	✓	✓				✓					✓	
Beets	✓		✓								✓								✓	
Broccoli	✓		✓	✓	✓		✓				✓	✓			✓	✓		✓	✓	✓
Brussels sprouts	✓		✓	✓							✓	✓			✓	✓		✓	✓	✓
Cabbage	✓		✓	✓								✓			✓	✓	✓	✓	✓	
Carrots	✓				✓	✓	✓				✓					✓	✓	✓	✓	
Cauliflower	✓		✓	✓		✓	✓				✓	✓		✓	✓	✓	✓	✓	✓	✓
Celery												✓			✓	✓		✓	✓	
Chickpeas			✓																	
Corn	✓		✓		✓		✓									✓	✓		✓	✓
Cucumber												✓				✓	✓			
Garlic	✓																	✓	✓	✓
Kale	✓	✓	✓	✓	✓		✓				✓				✓	✓		✓	✓	
Lentils		✓		✓	✓		✓				✓					✓	✓			
Mushrooms				✓	✓	✓					✓	✓					✓			
Onions	✓											✓								
Peas	✓	✓	✓	✓	✓	✓	✓			✓	✓	✓		✓		✓	✓		✓	
Peppers, sweet												✓	✓					✓		✓
Plantains	✓						✓									✓				
Potatoes					✓											✓			✓	✓
Pumpkin/Squash	✓															✓			✓	✓

DIETARY SOURCES OF VITAMINS AND MINERALS (CONTINUED)

FOOD SOURCES	Vit. A	Vit. B	Vit. B1	Vit. B2	Vit. B3	Vit. B5	Vit. B6	Vit. B12	Biotin	Choline	Folic Acid	Vit. C	Bioflavonoids	Vit. E	Vit. K	Iron	Zinc	Calcium	Magnesium	Potassium
Radishes	✓											✓								
Spinach	✓	✓	✓	✓							✓	✓		✓	✓	✓	✓	✓	✓	✓
Sweet potatoes	✓					✓					✓			✓						✓
Tomatoes												✓				✓				
Turnips											✓						✓	✓		
Watercress	✓		✓	✓			✓					✓			✓	✓		✓	✓	
Yams														✓	✓				✓	✓
Fruits (general)																				
Apples	✓			✓								✓				✓		✓	✓	
Apricots	✓												✓						✓	✓
Bananas							✓													✓
Blackberries												✓		✓		✓			✓	
Black currants												✓	✓			✓		✓	✓	
Cantaloupe/melons	✓						✓				✓									
Cherries	✓											✓	✓						✓	
Grapefruits	✓			✓								✓	✓							✓
Grapes													✓			✓				
Guavas												✓	✓							
Kiwis												✓								
Lemons												✓	✓						✓	✓
Mangoes	✓				✓							✓	✓			✓			✓	
Oranges	✓				✓						✓	✓	✓						✓	✓
Papayas	✓											✓						✓		✓
Peaches	✓											✓				✓		✓	✓	
Pears	✓											✓				✓		✓		
Pineapples	✓											✓							✓	
Plums	✓		✓											✓						✓
Strawberries	✓											✓								
Dried Fruits (general)																				
Apricots	✓																			✓
Currants				✓	✓						✓					✓		✓		✓
Dates	✓																	✓		✓

FOOD SOURCES	Vit. A	Vit. B	Vit. B₁	Vit. B₂	Vit. B₃	Vit. B₅	Vit. B₆	Vit. B₁₂	Biotin	Choline	Folic Acid	Vit. C	Bioflavonoids	Vit. E	Vit. K	Iron	Zinc	Calcium	Magnesium	Potassium
Figs																		✓	✓	✓
Prunes	✓		✓										✓			✓		✓	✓	✓
Raisins			✓													✓		✓	✓	✓
Nuts (general)			✓	✓		✓								✓		✓	✓	✓	✓	✓
Almonds				✓										✓		✓	✓	✓	✓	
Brazil nuts																✓		✓		
Cashews																✓		✓		
Hazelnuts							✓										✓			
Peanuts		✓	✓		✓		✓							✓		✓	✓	✓	✓	✓
Pecans		✓														✓	✓		✓	✓
Walnuts		✓					✓													
Seeds (general)																	✓			
Flaxseeds		✓	✓	✓	✓	✓	✓	✓						✓		✓	✓		✓	✓
Pumpkin seeds														✓		✓	✓	✓		
Sesame seeds														✓		✓		✓	✓	
Sunflower seeds							✓							✓		✓			✓	
Grains, whole (general)	✓				✓	✓					✓								✓	
Barley					✓															
Buckwheat					✓						✓		✓				✓		✓	
Cornmeal														✓					✓	
Millet														✓		✓				
Oatmeal			✓		✓										✓	✓				
Oats			✓		✓										✓	✓				
Rice bran							✓													
Rice, brown			✓			✓	✓				✓			✓		✓				✓
Rice, white						✓	✓													✓
Rye			✓		✓										✓	✓				
Wheat germ			✓	✓	✓	✓			✓	✓	✓						✓	✓	✓	✓
Wheat		✓	✓	✓	✓	✓			✓									✓	✓	
Miscellaneous																				
Brewer's yeast		✓	✓		✓				✓		✓					✓		✓	✓	✓
Corn flour			✓		✓									✓				✓	✓	
Dulce (seaweed)			✓	✓				✓				✓				✓		✓	✓	✓

DIETARY SOURCES OF VITAMINS AND MINERALS (CONTINUED)

FOOD SOURCES	Vit. A	Vit. B	Vit. B1	Vit. B2	Vit. B3	Vit. B5	Vit. B6	Vit. B12	Biotin	Choline	Folic Acid	Vit. C	Bioflavonoids	Vit. E	Vit. K	Iron	Zinc	Calcium	Magnesium	Potassium
Honey	✓																		✓	
Kelp			✓	✓	✓			✓				✓		✓	✓	✓	✓	✓	✓	
Molasses, blacktrap			✓	✓		✓									✓	✓	✓	✓	✓	✓
Olives																✓				
Royal jelly						✓														
Spirulina			✓																	
Tofu																✓		✓	✓	
Herbs and spices																				
Alfa alfa	✓		✓	✓	✓		✓	✓				✓		✓	✓	✓	✓	✓	✓	
Cayenne	✓		✓	✓	✓							✓				✓	✓	✓	✓	
Chamomile			✓	✓	✓											✓		✓	✓	
Chickweed	✓		✓	✓	✓							✓				✓		✓	✓	
Dandelion leaves	✓			✓	✓			✓				✓								
Elderberries													✓							
Fennel (seed)			✓	✓	✓							✓		✓		✓	✓	✓	✓	
Fenugreek			✓	✓	✓							✓				✓			✓	
Ginger					✓															
Ginseng				✓																
Lemongrass	✓																			
Licorice					✓		✓									✓			✓	
Marshmallow	✓		✓		✓									✓			✓	✓		✓
Nettle	✓			✓								✓				✓		✓	✓	
Paprika	✓		✓	✓	✓							✓				✓			✓	
Parsley	✓		✓	✓	✓							✓				✓		✓	✓	
Peppermint	✓		✓	✓								✓		✓		✓		✓		
Rose hips	✓		✓	✓								✓		✓		✓		✓		
Saffron	✓		✓	✓													✓		✓	
Sage	✓				✓															✓

YOUR FOOD DIARY

The food diary can be used to record your entire food and drink intake. The charts included on the pages that follow are sufficient for four weeks. You may wish to photocopy them (before writing on them) for use over a longer period of time. If you note on the charts the days of your period, you may find that you eat certain foods at a particular time in relation to your menstrual cycle. If you use the charts to note any physical symptoms, such as abdominal pain, you may find that it follows your intake of wheat, for example, and this could indicate that you have an allergy to it.

Use the charts to highlight the food groups, coding them by color as outlined below. This way, you will more clearly see whether you are consuming enough of the "Color 1" ("live") foods, and this may make it easier to change your eating habits. To code the foods you eat, you will need four highlighting pens of different colors. Highlight your food diary as follows:

Color 1: "Live" foods, including fruit, vegetables, pulses, whole grains (excluding wheat), seeds, nuts, oils, eggs, herbs, spices, fish, and organic poultry and meat.

Color 2: Foods that contain wheat, such as bread, cakes, cookies, and so on.

Color 3: Foods that contain dairy products, such as milk, cream, butter, cheese, yogurt, ice cream, sauces, and so on.

Color 4: Processed foods: canned, packaged, frozen, and chilled ready meals.

WEEK 1	Breakfast and drink	Mid-morning snack and/or drink	Lunch and drink	Mid-afternoon snack and/or drink	Evening meal and drink	Late snacks or drinks
Sunday						
Monday						
Tuesday						
Wednesday						
Thursday						
Friday						
Saturday						

WEEK 2	Breakfast and drink	Mid-morning snack and/or drink	Lunch and drink	Mid-afternoon snack and/or drink	Evening meal and drink	Late snacks or drinks
Sunday						
Monday						
Tuesday						
Wednesday						
Thursday						
Friday						
Saturday						

WEEK 3	Breakfast and drink	Mid-morning snack and/or drink	Lunch and drink	Mid-afternoon snack and/or drink	Evening meal and drink	Late snacks or drinks
Sunday						
Monday						
Tuesday						
Wednesday						
Thursday						
Friday						
Saturday						

WEEK 4	Breakfast and drink	Mid-morning snack and/or drink	Lunch and drink	Mid-afternoon snack and/or drink	Evening meal and drink	Late snacks or drinks
Sunday						
Monday						
Tuesday						
Wednesday						
Thursday						
Friday						
Saturday						

CHAPTER ELEVEN

Endo Data Files

Please complete the following questionnaires as honestly and as thoroughly as possible. This will enable you to assess your current lifestyle and allow your primary care provider, physician, or consultant to gain a wider perspective on your individual circumstances.

Either write in the answer or circle the response that is most appropriate to you. Not all the questions will be applicable to you; when one is not, please write "n/a."

1. PERSONAL DETAILS

Date:

Name:

Age:

Height:

Weight:

Address:

Zip or Postal code:

Telephone number(s):

Email address:

Marital Status

❑ Single ❑ Cohabiting ❑ Married ❑ Divorced ❑ Widowed

Occupation/profession
☐ Full-time ☐ Part-time ☐ Two jobs
What kind of work do you do? Please give details.

Do you think you might have endometriosis?
If so, who or what suggested this to you?
☐ Doctor ☐ Friend ☐ Book or magazine ☐ Website

Have you been given a definite diagnosis of endometriosis?
If so, by which method?
☐ Consultation ☐ Examination
☐ As a result of a surgical procedure ☐ Laparoscopy

When were you diagnosed with endometriosis?
Where?
By whom?

How old were you when diagnosed with endometriosis?

How long did it take after the start of your symptoms to get a diagnosis of endometriosis?
_____ years and _____ months

Please detail everything you know about your diagnosis, for example: What is your stage of endometriosis: 1, 2, 3, or 4?

What type of implants or cysts do you have?

Have adhesions been diagnosed?

Have you ever been diagnosed with any of the following?
☐ Polycystic ovaries ☐ Fibroids ☐ Ovarian cysts

Medical History

Have you ever suffered from any of the following?   *If so, when?*

Acne ❑ _____

Adenomyosis ❑ _____

Anemia ❑ _____

Asthma ❑ _____

Autoimmune disease (please detail) ❑ _____

Back pain ❑ _____

Bladder infection ❑ _____

Blood pressure: high ❑ _____

                low ❑ _____

Cancer or precancerous cells (please detail) ❑ _____

Candida, or yeast infection ❑ _____

Cystitis ❑ _____

Diabetes (please detail) ❑ _____

Eating disorder (please detail) ❑ _____

Eczema ❑ _____

Epilepsy ❑ _____

Fibromyalgia ❑ _____

Hay fever ❑ _____

Headache ❑ _____

Heart disease (please detail) ❑ _____

Herpes ❑ _____

Interstitial cystitis ❑ _____

Irritable bowel syndrome ❑ _____

Kidney problems (please detail) ❑ _____

Lupus ❑ _____

Migraine ❑ _____

Multiple sclerosis ❑ _____

Osteoporosis ❑ _____

Pelvic inflammatory disease ❑ _____

Premenstrual syndrome ❑ _____

Psoriasis ❑ _____

Sexually transmitted disease (please detail) ❑ _____

Thyroid problems (please detail) ❑ _____

Urinary tract infection ❑ _____

Urticaria ❑ _____

If you have, or have had, conditions not listed above, please list them in the appropriate section below (if you had these in the past, note how many years ago).

Cardiovascular:

Circulatory system:

Digestive system:

Endocrine system:

Immune system:

Musculoskeletal system:

Nervous system:

Respiratory system:

Skin:

Urinary system:

Other:

Medications and Prescription Drugs

Please list all prescribed medications you are taking at the present time.

Please list all prescribed medications you have taken in the past, and include the dates.

> Please also complete Endo Data Files 3 (page 233), 4 (page 236), and 5 (page 240), which detail any nutritional supplements you have taken, self-help treatments you have carried out, and treatments you have received from professional complementary-medicine practitioners.

Please detail any surgical procedures you have undergone, including laparoscopy, and include their dates.

Please detail nonprescription medication you have taken in the past, and include the dates.

Habits

Do you smoke?   How many cigarettes per day?

How many years have you been smoking?

If you have given up smoking, how many cigarettes did you smoke per day?

And for how many years?

When did you give them up?

Do you drink alcohol?   Approximate amount per week?

Do you drink any products that contain caffeine?
Approximate amount per week?

Lifestyle

Do you exercise regularly?

If so, how many times a week?   For how long?

What type of exercise do you do?

Do you engage in any other physical activity, such as dance or sports? Please detail.

Contraception

If you are sexually active, which contraceptive method are you currently using?

How long have you been using this method?

If you do not at present take the contraceptive pill, have you taken it in the past?

How many years did you take it, and when?

Early Menstrual History

At what age did you have your first period?

Were your periods heavy, light, or moderate?

Were they regular?   How long was a cycle?

How many days did your periods last?

Did you experience the following?
❑ Cramps ❑ Pain ❑ Nausea/vomiting ❑ Headaches ❑ Backache

What did you, or your parent or caregiver, do to ease them?

Did you visit a physician?

Please describe your parent's or caregiver's attitude to your periods.

Current Menstrual History

When did you first suspect there might be a problem with your menstrual cycle and periods?

On average, how many days are there between the start of one period and the next?

How many days does the bleeding last?

Do you consider your periods to be heavy, average, or light?

Do you pass any clots?

Do you experience any of the following?
❏ Cramps ❏ Pain ❏ Nausea/vomiting ❏ Headaches ❏ Backache

What do you do to ease your symptoms?

Premenstrual

Check any of the following that you experience before your period.

❏ Anger   ❏ Headaches

❏ Anxiety   ❏ Insomnia

❏ Bloating   ❏ Irritability

❏ Cravings   ❏ Mood swings

❏ Depression   ❏ Palpitations

❏ Emotional sensitivity   ❏ Tender breasts

❏ Fatigue   ❏ Weight gain

❏ Flulike symptoms

Postmenstrual

Check any of the following that you experience after your period.

❏ Anxiety   ❏ Lack of confidence

❏ Depression   ❏ Mood swings

❏ Irritability   ❏ Nervousness

How long do these symptoms last?

Family History

Has anyone else in your family suffered from any of the following?		*If so, who?*
Endometriosis	❏	_____
Painful periods	❏	_____
Miscarriage	❏	_____
Infertility	❏	_____
Ovarian cysts	❏	_____
Uterine cancer	❏	_____
Ovarian cancer	❏	_____
Any other types of cancer (please detail)	❏	_____

Sexual Activity

Do you have a regular sexual partner?

Do you find intercourse painful?

Do you find particular sexual intercourse positions uncomfortable?

Pregnancy

Have you ever been pregnant?
If so, how many times?

Have you ever had a termination/abortion?
If so, how many, and at what age or ages?

Have you ever had a miscarriage?
If so, how many, and at what age or ages?

Have you ever had an ectopic pregnancy?
If so, how many, and at what age or ages?

How many pregnancies have gone to full term?

How old were you when you had your child or children?

At the time of conception, had you been diagnosed with endometriosis, or was it suspected that you had endometriosis?

Postnatal

Have your periods returned to their pre-pregnancy pattern?
If not, how have they changed?

As compared with before your pregnancy, indicate whether your symptoms of endometriosis are now (check one):
❑ The same ❑ Worse ❑ Improved

Fertility

If you have not conceived, have you been trying?
If so, for how long?

If conception appears to be a problem, have you sought help?
If yes, from whom?

Have you ever taken drug therapy designed to increase fertility?

Have you had in vitro fertilization treatment?

Have you had any surgical procedures relating to fertility?
If so, which ones, and when?

What was the outcome of these treatments?

2. CURRENT SYMPTOMS

It is always useful for any person involved in your diagnosis and treatment to know as much as possible about your current symptoms. Some of the physical and mental health indicators may seem irrelevant in regard to any potential diagnosis of endometriosis or to fuller analysis of its extent, but these aspects may provide professionals with a broader view of your particular circumstances.

Pain before, during, or after Menstruation

Check off any of the sections that describe the pain you experience. You may need to check off more than one. If any of these types of pain occur only at a particular point in your menstrual cycle, please note when.

- ❏ Chronic pelvic pain (ongoing)
- ❏ Intermittent pelvic pain (occasional, generalized)
- ❏ Intermittent pelvic pain (occasional, sharp)
- ❏ Lower pelvic pain (from buttocks to groin)
- ❏ Severe abdominal cramps
- ❏ Continual abdominal dull ache

Menstrual Irregularity

There is no one "type" of menstrual cycle related to endometriosis. Some women have menstrual cycles far longer than thirty-one days, with little bleeding, while others have menstrual cycles so short one menstrual period seems to run into the next. However, most women with endometriosis have periods that are irregular in some way. (Irregular is defined as not occurring on a regular basis over a twenty-eight-to-thirty-one-day cycle.) Please indicate which type of menstrual cycle best describes your own, and add any further information if you wish.

❏ Heavy bleeding

❏ Scant bleeding

❏ Almost continuous blood flow during the month

❏ A cycle of between forty and sixty days

❏ A cycle with an unpredictable onset and duration

❏ Menstrual flow has clots

Other Pain, Aches, and Soreness

Please note whether you have pain in the following areas. Indicate how much pain — on a scale of 1 to 5, with 5 being the most painful.

❏ Backache (especially before and during periods)

❏ In the coccyx (bottom of spine)

❏ In one or more joints

❏ In the front of one or both thighs

❏ Headaches

❏ In the chest area

❏ In the shoulder

❏ In the rib cage (left, right, or both)

❏ Under the rib cage

❏ In the rectum

❏ In the vagina when inserting a tampon

Sex- and Reproduction-Related Issues

Have you experienced any of the following? Give details if you wish.

❑ Pain during or after sexual intercourse

❑ Infertility

❑ Miscarriage

❑ Ectopic pregnancy

❑ Decreased sex drive

❑ Increased sex drive

Hormonal Imbalance or Changes

There are many physical and mental indications of hormonal imbalance or change. Check off any of the following that you experience, and give details if you wish.

❑ Hot flashes

❑ Excessive perspiration (indicate day or night)

❑ Tender breasts

❑ Premenstrual syndrome (PMS)

❑ Excess of facial or body hair

❑ Deepening voice

Sometimes the condition of the skin indicates a hormonal condition or change. Indicate whether you feel your skin has become particularly

❑ Dry

❑ Greasy

❑ Acne prone

Skin Condition

Check off any of the following that describe your skin or parts of your skin.

❏ Spotty

❏ Flaky

❏ Scaly

❏ Presence of psoriasis

❏ Presence of eczema

❏ Presence of pigment changes

❏ Wounds that take a long time to heal

Digestive

Check off any of the following that relate to your experience, and give details if you wish.

❏ Painful defecation

❏ Constipation (often because it hurts to pass stools)

❏ Rectal bleeding or blood in stools

❏ Diarrhea

❏ Fluid retention

❏ Abdominal bloating

❏ Abdominal bloating that is progressive over the course of the day

❏ Feeling of "fullness"

❑ Abdomen feels "lumpy"

❑ Pain on one side of abdomen (indicate which)

❑ Excessive gas

❑ Sharp gas pains

❑ Indigestion

❑ Nausea or vomiting

❑ Sugar cravings

❑ Loss of appetite

Urinary

Check off any sections that relate to your experience, and give details if you wish.

❑ Frequent urination

❑ Urgent urination

❑ Loss of control of urination

❑ Difficulty in passing urine

❑ Blood in urine

❑ Kidney tenderness

Cardiovascular

Check off any sections that relate to your experience, and give details if you wish.

❑ Palpitations

❑ Dizziness

❑ High blood pressure

❑ Breathlessness

Breathing

Do you sometimes have difficulty breathing?

Do you sometimes have pain in the abdomen when breathing deeply?

Mind, Mood, and Emotion

Do you experience any of the following, and if so, in what circumstances?

❑ Depression

❑ Anxiety

❑ Panic attacks

❑ Nervousness

❑ Irritability

❑ Poor concentration

❑ Poor memory

❑ Confusion

❑ Difficulty making decisions

❑ Loss of confidence

❑ Loss of vitality

❑ Apathy

❏ Fatigue

❏ Exhaustion

❏ Insomnia

Body Temperature

Body temperature can indicate changes in different physical systems, particularly the hormonal system or nervous system.

Do you feel cold all the time?

Do you alternate between feeling hot and cold?

Do you feel very cold in your hands or feet? If so, which?

Nerves

Do you experience any of the following? If so, describe where and how often.

❏ Numbness in your back

❏ Numbness in your fingers or hands

❏ Numbness in your toes or feet

❏ Numbness in one or both arms (which?)

❏ Numbness in your legs

❏ Tingling in your fingers or hands

❏ Tingling in your toes or feet

❏ Tingling in your legs

3. NUTRITIONAL SUPPLEMENTS

Please list any supplements that you take, detailing the dosages or number of tablets or capsules and the time or times of day. If you take complex mixes of supplements, attach to this questionnaire a detailed list or a label from the bottle. If you know whether the supplement is from a natural or synthetic source, please indicate this also.

Vitamins

<u>Vitamin 1</u>
Vitamin name: ❑ Natural   or   ❑ Synthetic
Dosage per day:
Times of day you take it (check all that apply):
    ❑ Morning ❑ Afternoon ❑ Evening
Regularity: ❑ Consistently ❑ Infrequently or when I remember

<u>Vitamin 2</u>
Vitamin name: ❑ Natural   or   ❑ Synthetic
Dosage per day:
Times of day you take it (check all that apply):
    ❑ Morning ❑ Afternoon ❑ Evening
Regularity: ❑ Consistently ❑ Infrequently or when I remember

<u>Vitamin 3</u>
Vitamin name: ❑ Natural   or   ❑ Synthetic
Dosage per day:
Times of day you take it (check all that apply):
    ❑ Morning ❑ Afternoon ❑ Evening
Regularity: ❑ Consistently ❑ Infrequently or when I remember

Minerals

<u>Mineral 1</u>
Mineral name: ❑ Natural   or   ❑ Synthetic

Dosage per day:

Times of day you take it (check all that apply):

    ❑ Morning ❑ Afternoon ❑ Evening

Regularity: ❑ Consistently ❑ Infrequently or when I remember

Mineral 2

Mineral name: ❑ Natural or ❑ Synthetic

Dosage per day:

Times of day you take it (check all that apply):

    ❑ Morning ❑ Afternoon ❑ Evening

Regularity: ❑ Consistently ❑ Infrequently or when I remember

Trace Elements

Trace Element 1

Trace Element name: ❑ Natural or ❑ Synthetic

Dosage per day:

Times of day you take it (check all that apply):

    ❑ Morning ❑ Afternoon ❑ Evening

Regularity: ❑ Consistently ❑ Infrequently or when I remember

Trace Element 2

Trace Element name: ❑ Natural or ❑ Synthetic

Dosage per day:

Times of day you take it (check all that apply):

    ❑ Morning ❑ Afternoon ❑ Evening

Regularity: ❑ Consistently ❑ Infrequently or when I remember

Amino Acids

Amino Acid 1

Amino Acid name: ❑ Natural or ❑ Synthetic

Dosage per day:

Times of day you take it (check all that apply):

    ❑ Morning ❑ Afternoon ❑ Evening

Regularity: ❑ Consistently ❑ Infrequently or when I remember

Amino Acid 2

Amino Acid name: ❏ Natural or ❏ Synthetic

Dosage per day:

Times of day you take it (check all that apply):

    ❏ Morning ❏ Afternoon ❏ Evening

Regularity: ❏ Consistently ❏ Infrequently or when I remember

Esssential Fatty Acids/Oils

Essentail Fatty Acid/Oil 1

Oil name: ❏ Natural or ❏ Synthetic

Dosage per day:

Times of day you take it (check all that apply):

    ❏ Morning ❏ Afternoon ❏ Evening

Regularity: ❏ Consistently ❏ Infrequently or when I remember

Essentail Fatty Acid/Oil 2

Oil name: ❏ Natural or ❏ Synthetic

Dosage per day:

Times of day you take it (check all that apply):

    ❏ Morning ❏ Afternoon ❏ Evening

Regularity: ❏ Consistently ❏ Infrequently or when I remember

Other

Other Supplement 1

Supplement name: ❏ Natural or ❏ Synthetic

Dosage per day:

Times of day you take it (check all that apply):

    ❏ Morning ❏ Afternoon ❏ Evening

Regularity: ❏ Consistently ❏ Infrequently or when I remember

Other Supplement 2

Supplement name: ❏ Natural or ❏ Synthetic

Dosage per day:

Times of day you take it (check all that apply):

    ❏ Morning ❏ Afternoon ❏ Evening

Regularity: ❏ Consistently ❏ Infrequently or when I remember

4. SELF-TREATMENT

Have you been using natural remedies to treat yourself, either for endometriosis or for another condition? If so, please complete the relevant section or sections below.

Herbal Remedies

Herb 1
Herb name:
Form (tincture, capsules, tea, etc.):
Dates of use: from _____ to _____
Frequency of use:
Reason for use: ❏ Endometriosis ❏ Another condition or reason
If another condition or reason, please specify:
Outcome or result of this treatment:

Herb 2
Herb name:
Form (tincture, capsules, tea, etc.):
Dates of use: from _____ to _____
Frequency of use:
Reason for use: ❏ Endometriosis ❏ Another condition or reason
If another condition or reason, please specify:
Outcome or result of this treatment:

Chinese Herbs

Chinese Herb 1
Chinese Herb name:

Form (tincture, capsules, tea, etc.):

Dates of use: from _____ to _____

Frequency of use:

Reason for use: ❑ Endometriosis ❑ Another condition or reason

If another condition or reason, please specify:

Outcome or result of this treatment:

Chinese Herb 2

Chinese Herb name:

Form (tincture, capsules, tea, etc.):

Dates of use: from _____ to _____

Frequency of use:

Reason for use: ❑ Endometriosis ❑ Another condition or reason

If another condition or reason, please specify:

Outcome or result of this treatment:

Essential Oils and Aromatherapy Oils

Essential Oil (or Oil Blend) 1

Name of oil(s):

Method (sitz bath, massage or bath oil, diffuser, etc.):

Amount used:

Dates of use: from _____ to _____

Frequency of use:

Reason for use: ❑ Endometriosis ❑ Another condition or reason

If another condition or reason, please specify:

Outcome or result of this treatment:

Essential Oil (or Oil Blend) 2

Name of oil(s):

Method (sitz bath, massage or bath oil, diffuser, etc.):

Amount used:

Dates of use: from _____ to _____

Frequency of use:

Reason for use: ❑ Endometriosis   ❑ Another condition or reason

If another condition or reason, please specify:

Outcome or result of this treatment:

Homeopathy

Homeopathic Remedy 1

Name of remedy:

Dates of use: from _____ to _____

Frequency of use:

Reason for use: ❑ Endometriosis   ❑ Another condition or reason

If another condition or reason, please specify: _____

Outcome or result of this treatment:

Homeopathic Remedy 2

Name of remedy:

Dates of use: from _____ to _____
Frequency of use:
Reason for use: ❑ Endometriosis ❑ Another condition or reason
If another condition or reason, please specify: _____
Outcome or result of this treatment:

Flower Remedies

Flower Remedy 1
Name of remedy:
Amount used:
Dates of use: from _____ to _____
Frequency of use:
Reason for use: ❑ Endometriosis ❑ Another condition or reason
If another condition or reason, please specify: _____
Outcome or result of this treatment:

Flower Remedy 2
Name of remedy:
Amount used:
Dates of use: from _____ to _____
Frequency of use:
Reason for use: ❑ Endometriosis ❑ Another condition or reason
If another condition or reason, please specify: _____
Outcome or result of this treatment:

5. PROFESSIONAL TREATMENT:
COMPLEMENTARY MEDICINE

Have you been treated by a professional practitioner in any of the following complementary therapies, either for endometriosis or for another condition? If so, please complete the relevant section or sections below.

Acupuncture

Dates of treatment: from _____ to _____
Reason for treatment: ❑ Endometriosis ❑ Another condition
If another condition, please specify:
Which areas did, or does, your practitioner concentrate on?

What was the outcome, or what has it been so far?

Chiropractic

Dates of treatment: from _____ to _____
Reason for treatment: ❑ Endometriosis ❑ Another condition
If another condition, please specify:
Which areas did, or does, your practitioner concentrate on?

What was the outcome, or what has it been so far?

Cranial Osteopathy

Dates of treatment: from _____ to _____
Reason for treatment: ❑ Endometriosis ❑ Another condition

If another condition, please specify:
Which areas did, or does, your practitioner concentrate on?

What was the outcome, or what has it been so far?

Massage

Types of massage:
Dates of treatment: from _____ to _____
Frequency of treatment:
Reason for treatment: ❑ Endometriosis ❑ Another condition
If another condition, please specify:
Which areas of the body did, or does, your practitioner concentrate on?

What was the outcome, or what has it been so far?

Osteopathy

Dates of treatment: from _____ to _____
Frequency of treatment:
Reason for treatment: ❑ Endometriosis ❑ Another condition
If another condition, please specify:
Which areas did, or does, your practitioner concentrate on?

What was the outcome, or what has it been so far?

Reflexology

Dates of treatment: from _____ to _____

Frequency of treatment:

Reason for treatment: ❏ Endometriosis   ❏ Another condition

If another condition, please specify:

Which areas did, or does, your practitioner concentrate on?

What was the outcome, or what has it been so far?

Reiki

Dates of treatment: from _____ to _____

Frequency of treatment:

Reason for treatment: ❏ Endometriosis   ❏ Another condition

If another condition, please specify:

Which areas did, or does, your practitioner concentrate on?

What was the outcome, or what has it been so far?

Shiatsu

Type of Shiatsu:

Dates of treatment: from _____ to _____

Frequency of treatment:

Reason for treatment: ❏ Endometriosis ❏ Another condition

If another condition or reason, please specify:

Which areas did, or does, your practitioner concentrate on?

What was the outcome, or what has it been so far?

Other Healing Modalities

Modality 1

Name of modality:

Dates of treatment: from _____ to _____

Frequency of treatment:

Reason for treatment: ❏ Endometriosis ❏ Another condition

If another condition or reason, please specify:

Which areas did, or does, your practitioner concentrate on?

What was the outcome, or what has it been so far?

Modality 2
Name of modality:
Dates of treatment: from _____ to _____
Frequency of treatment:
Reason for treatment: ❑ Endometriosis   ❑ Another condition
If another condition, please specify:
Which areas did, or does, your practitioner concentrate on?

What was the outcome, or what has it been so far?

Modality 3
Name of modality:
Dates of treatment: from _____ to _____
Frequency of treatment:
Reason for treatment: ❑ Endometriosis   ❑ Another condition
If another condition, please specify:
Which areas did, or does, your practitioner concentrate on?

What was the outcome, or what has it been so far?

Abdomen: the cavity between the diaphragm and pelvis; contains the stomach, intestines, liver, spleen, kidneys, pancreas, and, in women, the uterus, ovaries, and fallopian tubes.

Acute pain: temporary pain (see Chronic pain).

Adenomyosis: disease in which endometrial tissue grows inside the muscular walls of the uterus.

Adhesions: connective tissue joining two or more surfaces, which forms in response to inflammation or other tissue damage. (Fibrous adhesions: connective tissue containing fibers or resembling fibers.)

Aetiology: see Etiology.

Allopathic (medicine): also known as "conventional medicine"; treatment with pharmaceutical drugs and surgery.

Analgesics: drugs to ease pain.

Androgens: hormones produced in large quantity in male testes and in tiny quantities in ovaries and adrenal glands; drug treatment given to women with endometriosis to suppress reproductive tract activity.

Antibodies: specialist proteins created by the lymph system in response to substances harmful to the body.

ATP: adenosine triphosphate.

Autoimmune diseases: disorders caused by the incorrect working of the body's own cells or defense system of antibodies.

CAT (CT) scan: computed axial tomography; diagnostic procedure used to help identify the location of endometrial implants and adhesions.

CDI: color Doppler imaging.

Chronic pain: pain that continues for more than six months (see Acute pain).

Corpus luteum: sac in ovary containing the ovum, and which ruptures to release the ovum during ovulation.

CRP: C-reactive protein.

Culdocentesis: diagnostic procedure to remove fluid from pelvic cavity using a needle pressed through the vaginal wall.

Cyst: a sac filled with liquid or semisolid material.

Cystoscopy (or Cystourethroscopy): diagnostic procedure to view inside the urethra, ureters, and bladder using a thin fiberoptic tube.

Diffusers: equipment designed to release airborne aromatic molecules from essential oils.

DNA: deoxyribonucleic acid.

Dysmenorrhea: painful periods.

Dyspareunia: painful intercourse.

Dysuria: painful urination.

EBT: electron-beam tomography; diagnostic procedure used to help identify the location of endometrial implants and adhesions.

Endometrioma: cyst filled with old blood; often called "chocolate cyst."

Endometriosis interna: adenomyosis (see above).

ER-α: estrogen receptor alpha.

ER-ß: estrogen receptor beta.

Etiology: branch of medicine dealing with the cause of a disease.

Fallopian tubes: two tubes extending from the left and right sides of the upper uterus, in which ova are fertilized by sperm.

FSH: follicle-stimulating hormone.

GM: genetically modified or manipulated.

GnRH: gonadotropin-releasing hormone.

HDL: High-density lipoproteins.

Histogenesis: the development of tissue.

HRT: hormone replacement therapy.

Hysterectomy: surgical removal of the uterus and cervix.

Hysterectomy with bilateral salpingo-oophorectomy: surgical removal of the fallopian tubes and ovaries as well as the uterus and cervix.

Hysterosalpingography: diagnostic procedure to view inside the uterus and to ascertain, by means of x-ray imagery and dye injected into the uterus, whether the fallopian tubes are blocked.

Hysteroscopy: diagnostic procedure to view inside the uterus to determine, by means of a liquid or carbon dioxide gas to inflate the uterine cavity, and then a light-scope, whether adenomyosis nodules, fibroids, or polyps are present.

Implants, endometrial: endometrial cells that have implanted in tissue other than the interior lining of the uterus.

IVF: in vitro fertilization.

Laparoscope: instrument used in laparoscopy; thin tube with a camera and light attached, used to examine the abdominal cavity.

Laparoscopy: diagnostic procedure often used in conjunction with actual surgery to view inside the abdominal cavity by means of a thin tube (laparoscope) inserted through the abdomen. Carbon dioxide gas is first pumped into the cavity to separate internal organs and make viewing easier.

Laparotomy: surgical procedure in which a cut is made above the pubic hairline and the surgeon cuts, cauterizes, or vaporizes cysts, nodules, or endometrial implants. The surgeon may also perform other surgical procedures, such as the removal of ovaries.

LDL: low-density lipoproteins.

LH: luteinizing hormone.

Lignans: vegetable fiber with estrogenlike activity.

Menarche: the onset of menstruation.

MRI: magnetic resonance imaging; diagnostic procedure used to help identify the location of endometrial implants and adhesions.

Oophorectomy (or Ovariectomy): surgical procedure to remove the ovaries. (Unilateral oophorectomy: the removal of one ovary; bilateral oophorectomy: the removal of both ovaries.)

Ovaries: the two organs containing the ova.

Pathogenesis: the origin of a disease.

Peritoneum: membrane lining the abdominal cavity.

PID: pelvic inflammatory disease.

PMS: premenstrual syndrome.

Prognosis: expected development of a medical condition, based on current symptoms, and the medical treatment being given.

Prostaglandins: substances produced by the body that perform several functions, including the contraction and relaxation of smooth muscles.

Referred pain: also known as "antidromic pain"; pain felt in muscles, tissues, or skin whose source is actually in the internal organs.

Retrograde menstruation: the flow of menstrual fluid through one or both fallopian tubes and into the abdominal cavity, rather than through the cervix and vagina.

RNA: ribonucleic acid.

SERMs: selective estrogen receptor modulators.

Transdermal: through the skin.

Ultrasound (or Ultrasonography): diagnostic procedure using sound waves to create a visual image. Pelvic ultrasound or Transabdominal sonography: a transducer is applied to the abdomen; Vaginal ultrasound or Transvaginal ultrasonography (TVS): a transducer is introduced into the vagina.

Urethritis: inflammation of the urethra having several possible causes.

Uterosacral ligaments: ligaments joining uterus and sacrum.

Uterus: womb.

Visceral nerves: nerves supplying the uterus, fallopian tubes, ovaries, and all other internal organs.

An, Jinping, et al. 2001. "Estrogen Receptor B-Selective Transcriptional Activity and Recruitment of Coregulators by Phytoestrogens." *Journal of Biological Chemistry* 276:17808–14.

Aqel, M., and R. Shaheen. 1996. "Effects of the Volatile Oil of *Nigella sativa* Seeds on the Uterine Smooth Muscle of Rat and Guinea Pig." *Journal of Ethnopharmacology* 52:23–26.

Araujo, I. B., et al. 1996. "Study of the Embryofoetotoxicity of Alpha-Terpinene in the Rat." *Food and Chemical Toxicology* 34:477–82.

Bach, Edward. 2005. *The Essential Writings of Dr. Edward Bach*. New York: Random House.

Baerwald, Angela R., Gregg P. Adams, and Roger A. Pierson. 2003. "Characterization of Ovarian Follicular Wave Dynamics in Women." *Biology of Reproduction* 69:1023–31.

Ballweg, Mary Lou, and Susan Deutsch. 1988. *Overcoming Endometriosis*. London: Arlington Books.

Benzie, A. 1992. "Aromatherapy and Herbal Medicine vs PMT — Co-operative Venture." *International Journal of Complementary Medicine* 10:25.

Brosens, Jan J. 1998. "Steroid Hormone-Dependent Myometrial Zonal Differentiation in the Non-pregnant Human Uterus." *European Journal of Obstetrics and Gynecology* 81:247–51.

Bulun, S. E., E. Serdar, et al. 2000. "Aromatase as a Therapeutic Target in Endometriosis." *Trends in Endocrinology and Metabolism* 11:1.

Bulun, S. E., K. M. Zeitoun, et al. 2002. "Expression of Dioxin-Related Transactivating Factors and Target Genes in Human Genes in Human Eutopic Endometrial and Endometriotic Tissues." *American Journal of Obstetrics and Gynecology* 182:767–75.

Butler, E. B., and E. McKnight. 1995. "Vitamin E in the Treatment of Primary Dysmenorrhoea." *Lancet* 1:844–47.

Cai, L. 1999. "Clinical and Experimental Study on the Treatment of Endometriosis with Dan'e Mixture." *Zhongguo Zhong Xi Yi Jie He Za Zhi* 19:159–61.

Canavan, Timothy P., and Lee Radosh. 2000. "Managing Endometriosis: Strategies to Minimize Pain and Damage." *Postgraduate Medicine* 107:3.

Chan, Kelvin, and Lily Cheung. 2000. *Interactions between Chinese Herbal Medicinal Products and Orthodox Drugs.* London: Taylor and Francis Group.

Charman, D. L. 1976. "Endometriosis in the Black Woman." *American Journal of Obstetrics and Gynecology* 125:596–601.

Child, T. J., and S. L. Tan. 2001. "Endometriosis: Aetiology, Pathogenesis, and Treatment." *Drugs* 61:1735–50.

Darbre, P. D., et al. 2004. "Concentrations of Parabens in Human Breast Tumours." *Journal of Applied Toxicology* 24:5–13.

D'Hooghe, T. M., et al. 2002. "Endometriosis, Retrograde Menstruation, and Peritoneal Inflammation in Women and in Baboons." *Human Reproduction Update* 8:84–88.

———. 1999. "Pelvic Inflammation Induced by Diagnostic Laparoscopy in Baboons." *Fertility and Sterility* 72:1134–41.

———. 1996. "Development of Spontaneous Endometriosis in Baboons." *Obstetrics and Gynecology* 88:462–66.

———. 1996. "Effect of Endometriosis on White Blood Cell Subpopulations in Peripheral Blood and Peritoneal Fluid on Baboons." *Human Reproduction* 11:1736–40.

———. 1996. "Increased Prevalence and Recurrence of Retrograde Menstruation in Baboons with Spontaneous Endometriosis." *Human Reproduction* 11:2022–25.

———. 1995. "The Effects of Immunosuppression on Development and Progression of Endometriosis in Baboons (Papio anubis)." *Fertility and Sterility* 64:172–78.

Elder, R. L. 1984. "Final Report on the Safety Assessment of Methylparaben, Ethylparaben, Propylparaben and Butylparaben." *Journal of the American College of Toxicology* 3:147–209.

EU Commission. "Strategy for a Future Chemicals Policy — REACH" White Paper, COM (2001) 0088 final. February 27, 2007.

Farquhar, C. 2001. "Endometriosis." *Clinical Evidence* 7:1654–62.

Farquhar, C., and C. Sutton. 1998. "The Evidence for the Management of Endometriosis." *Current Opinion in Obstetrics and Gynaecology* 10:321–32.

Flaws, Bob. 1989. *Endometriosis, Infertility, and Traditional Chinese Medicine.* Boulder: Blue Poppy Books.

Fontana, Aurelie, and Pierre Delmas. 2001. "Clinical Use of Selective Estrogen Receptor Modulators." *Current Opinion in Rheumatology* 13(4):333–39.

Glenville, Marilyn. 2001. *The Nutritional Health Handbook for Women.* London: Judy Piatkus.

Gokhale, L. B. 1996. "Curative Treatment of Primary (Spasmodic) Dysmenorrhoea." *Indian Journal of Medical Research* 103:227–31.

Grant, Ellen. 1994. *Sexual Chemistry.* Reading, U.K.

Hall, Julie M., and Kenneth S. Korach. 2002. "Analysis of the Molecular Mechanisms of Human Estrogen Receptors a and b Reveals Differential Specificity in Target Promoter Regulation by Xenoestrogens." *Journal of Biological Chemistry* 277:44455–61.

Halstead, L., P. Pepping, and W. P. Dmowski. 1989. "The Woman with Endometriosis: Dismissed, Devalued, Ignored." *Second International Symposium on Endometriosis*, Houston, TX, May 13, 1989.

Hammer, K. A., et al. 1998. "In-Vitro Activity of Essential Oils, in Particular Melaleuca alternifolia (Tea Tree) Oil and Tea Tree Oil Products, against Candida spp." *Journal of Antimicrobial Chemotherapy* 42:591–95.

Harvey, Philip W., and David J. Everett. 2004. "Editorial: Significance of the Detection of Esters of p-Hydroxybenzoic Acid (Parabens) in Human Breast Tumours." *Journal of Applied Toxicology* 24:1–4.

Henry, John A., ed. 1997. *British Medical Association: The New Guide to Medicine and Drugs.* London: Dorling Kindersley.

Hufnagel, Vicki. 1989. *No More Hysterectomies.* New York: Plume.

Hughes, E., et al. 2003. "Ovulation Suppression for Endometriosis." *Cochrane Database of Systematic Reviews*, Issue 3. Art. No.: CD000155. DOI: 10.1002/14651858.CD000155.

Ibarra, R. 1997. "Chronobiology and the Homeopathic Treatment of Menstrual Disorders." *Homeopath International* 11:26–27.

Jarry, H., et al. 2003. "In Vitro Effects of the *Cimicifuga racemosa* Extract BNO 1055." *Maturitas* 44, suppl. 1:31–38.

Jori, A., et al. 1970. "Effect of Eucalyptol (1,8-cineole) on the Metabolism of Other Drugs in Rats and in Man." *European Journal of Pharmacology* 9:362–66.

Kats, R., et al. 2002. "Marked Elevation of Macrophage Migration Inhibitory Factor in the Peritoneal Fluid of Women with Endometriosis." *Fertility and Sterility* 78:69–76.

Kennedy, S. 1998. "The Genetics of Endometriosis." *Journal of Reproductive Medicine* 43, suppl.:263–68.

Koninckx, P. R., et al. 1992. "CA-125 and Placental Protein 14 Concentrations in Plasma and Peritoneal Fluid of Women with Deeply Infiltrating Pelvic Endometriosis." *Fertility and Sterility* 57:523–30.

Lavery, S. 1994. "Aromatherapy Saved Me from a Hysterectomy." *Here's Health* 12:65–66.

Lieberman, S. 1998. "A Review of the Effectiveness of *Cimicifuga racemosa* (Black Cohosh) for the Symptoms of Menopause." *Journal of Women's Health* 7:525–29.

Lis-Balchnin, Maria. 2002. *Geranium and Pelargonium*. London: Taylor and Francis.

Lithgow, D., and W. Politzer. 1977. "Vitamin A in the Treatment of Menorrhagia." *South African Medical Journal* 51:191–93.

Liu, J. X. 1998. "Clinical Observations on Treatment of Endometriosis by Tonifying Kidney and Removing Blood Statis." *Zhongguo Zhong Xi Yi Jie He Za Zhi* 18:145–47.

———. 1994. "Clinical Study of the Treatment of Endometriosis with Traditional Chinese Medicine." *Chung Kuo Chung Hsi I Chieh Ho Tsa Chih* 14:323–24, 337–39.

Mathias, J. R., et al. 1998. "Relation of Endometriosis and Neuromuscular Disease of the Gastrointestinal Tract: New Insights." *Fertility and Sterility* 70:81–88.

McCormack, E. 2000. "Aromatherapy and Treatment of the Reproductive System." *Aromatic News* 3–6, Winter.

Meggs, William Joel. 2003. *The Inflammation Cure*. New York: Contemporary Books.

Moore, J., et al. 1997. "Modern Combined Oral Contraceptives for Pain Associated with Endometriosis." *Cochrane Database of Systematic Reviews* 1997, Issue 4. Art. No.: CD001019. DOI: 10.1002/14651858.CD001019.

Mori, M., et al. 2002. "Quality Evaluation of Essential Oils." *Yakugaku Zasshi* 122:253–61.

Mori, T., et al. 1993. "Suppression of Spontaneous Development of Uterine Adenomyosis by a Chinese Herbal Medicine, Keishi-buuryo-gan, in Mice." *Planta Medica* 59:308–11.

Nissim, Rina. 1986. *Natural Healing in Gynecology*. New York: Pandora.

Nwodo, O. F. 1991. "Studies on *Abrus precatorius* Seeds. 1. Uterotonic Activity of Seed Oil." *Journal of Ethnopharmacology* 31:391–93.

Oliker, A. J., and A. E. Harries. 1971. "Endometriosis of the Bladder in a Male Patient." *Journal of Urology* 106:858.

Paumgartten, F. J., et al. 1998. "Study of the Effects of Beta-Myrcene on Rat Fertility and General Reproductive Performance." *Brazilian Journal of Medical and Biological Research* 31:955–65.

Pert, Candace B. 1997. *Molecules of Emotion.* New York: Simon and Schuster.

Phipps, W. R., et al. 1993. "Effect of Flax Seed Ingestion on the Menstrual Cycle." *Journal of Clinical Endocrinology and Metabolism* 77:1215–19.

Pierson R. A., et al. 2003. "Characterization of Ovarian Follicular Wave Dynamics in Women." *Biology of Reproduction* 69:1023–31.

Rastogi, S. C., et al. 1995. "Contents of Methyl-, Ethyl-, Propyl-, Butyl- and Benzylparaben in Cosmetic Products." *Contact Dermatitis* 32:28–30.

Renner, S. P., et al. 2006. "Evaluation of Clinical Parameters and Estrogen Receptor Alpha Gene Polymorphisms for Patients with Endometriosis." *Reproduction* 131:153–61.

Rice, V. M. 2002. "Conventional Medical Therapies for Endometriosis." *Annals of the New York Academy of Sciences* 955:343–52.

Rudel, R. A., et al. 2003. "Phthalates, Alkylphenols, Pesticides, Polybrominated Diphenyl Ethers, and Other Endocrine-Disrupting Compounds Indoor Air and Dust." *Environmental Science and Technology* 37 (20): 4543–53.

Sampson, J. A. 1927. "Peritoneal Endometriosis Due to the Menstrual Dissemination of Endometrial Tissue into the Peritoneal Cavity." *American Journal of Obstetrics and Gynecology* 14:422–25.

Santillo, David, et al. 2003. "Consuming Chemicals: Hazardous Chemicals in House Dust as an Indicator of Chemical Exposure in the Home: Part I — UK." *Greenpeace Research Laboratories Technical Note* 01/2003.

———. 2003. "Hazardous Chemicals in House Dusts as an Indicator of Chemical Exposure in the Home: Part II — Germany, Spain, Slovakia, Italy and France." *Greenpeace Research Laboratories Technical Note* 02/2003.

Schellenberg, R. 2001. "Treatment for the Premenstrual Syndrome with Agnus Castus Fruit Extract: Prospective, Randomised Placebo-Controlled Study." *British Medical Journal* 322:134–37.

Schuessler, W. H. 1970. *The Biochemic Handbook.* Rev. ed. London: New Era Laboratories.

Selak, V., et al. 2001. "Danazol for Pelvic Pain Associated with Endometriosis." *Cochrane Database of Systematic Reviews* 2001, Issue 4. Art. No.: CD000068. DOI: 10.1002/14651858.CD000068.

Sharpe, R. M., and D. S. Irvine. 2004. "How Strong Is the Evidence of a Link Between Environmental Chemicals and Adverse Effects on Human Reproductive Health?" *British Medical Journal* 328:447–51.

Sinaii, N., S. D. Cleary, M. L. Ballweg, L. K. Niewman, and P. Stratton. 2002. "High Rates of Autoimmune and Endocrine Disorders, Fibromyalgia, Chronic Fatigue Syndrome, and Atopic Diseases among Women with Endometriosis: A Survey Analysis." *Human Reproduction* 17:2715–24.

Society of Homeopaths (United Kingdom). n.d. "Past, Present, and Future Medicine." Available at http://www.homeopathy-soh.org/about-homeopathy /what-is-homeopathy/past-present-and-future.aspx.

Suresh, B., et al. 1997. "Anticandidal Activity of *Santolina chamaecyparissus* Volatile Oil." *Journal of Ethnopharmacology* 55:151–59.

Svigos, J. 1990. Letter to the editor. *British Medical Journal.* February 24, 1990.

Tanaka, T., et al. 1998. "A Preliminary Immunopharmacological Study of an Antiendometriotic Herbal Medicine, Keishi-bukaryo-gan." *Osaka City Medical Journal* 44:117–24.

Torii S., et al. 1988. "Contingent Negative Variation (CNV) and the Psychological Effects of Odor." In *Perfumery: The Psychology and Biology of Fragrance,* edited by Steve Van Toller and George H. Dodd, 107–46. London and New York: Chapman and Hall.

Trickey, R. 1995. "A Look at the Herbal Treatment of Excess Menstruation: Past and Present." *Australian Journal of Medical Herbalism* 7:85–94.

Uphof, J. C. T. 1968. *Dictionary of Economic Plants.* Lehre: Verlag von J. Cramer.

Waterland, R. A., and R. L. Jirtle. 2003. "Transposable Elements: Targets for Early Nutritional Effects on Epigenetic Gene Regulation." *Molecular and Cellular Biology* 23:5293–300.

Winkel, C. A., and A. R. Scialli. 2001. "Medical and Surgical Therapies for Pain Associated with Endometriosis." *Journal of Women's Health and Gender-Based Medicine* 10:137–62.

Witz, C. A. 2002. "Pathogenesis of Endometriosis." *Gynecology and Obstetric Investigation* 53, suppl:1:52–62.

World Wildlife Fund. "Living Planet Report 2004." October 21, 2004. Available at http://www.worldwildlife.org/about/lpr2004.pdf.

Worwood, Valerie Ann. 2003. *Essential Aromatherapy.* Novato, CA: New World Library.

———. 2001. *Aromatherapy for the Beauty Therapist.* London: Thomson Learning.

———. 1999. *Aromatherapy for the Soul.* Novato, CA: New World Library.

———. 1996. *The Fragrant Mind.* Novato, CA: New World Library.

———. 1991. *The Complete Book of Essential Oils and Aromatherapy.* Novato, CA: New World Library.

MEASUREMENT CONVERSIONS:
METRIC AND IMPERIAL

1 milliliter (ml) = 0.033814 fluid ounces (USA liquid)
= 0.0351951 fluid ounces (UK liquid)

Metric		Imperial
30 ml	=	1 fl oz
15 ml	=	1/2 fl oz
10 ml	=	1/3 fl oz
5 ml	=	1/6 fl oz

TREATMENT PLAN SUPPLIES

Natural organic products, including organic essential oils, herbs, and nutritional supplements, can be purchased from good health food shops and specialist suppliers.

A recommended supplier of essential oils in Europe is:

Earth Garden
2 Fairview Parade, Mawney Road
Romford RM7 7HH
Essex, United Kingdom
00 (44) 1708 722633
www.earthgarden.co.uk

Or
For essential oils and organic products, visit
www.valerieworwood.com

Page numbers in italics refer to illustrations.

A

acupuncture and acupressure, 126, 133–35
adenomyosis, 18–19; CDI for diagnosis, 15, 19; Chinese herbs for, 129–30; as disease of the cells, 36–39; hysteroscopy for diagnosis, 16; symptoms similar to endometriosis, 17, 18
adhesions: exercise for, 66; in moderate to severe endometriosis, 4–5; pain and, 5, 8; pelvic, 16; resulting from surgery, 43
adrenal hormones: vitamin B needs, 178; vitamin B_5 for, 181
affirmations, 50–51
Agnus castus. *See* chaste berry (*Vitex agnus castus*)
alcohol: cell damage and, 39; elimination of intake of, 105, 110, 119; liver function and, 53–54, 55; vitamin B deficiency and, 179, 180
aloe vera juice, 99
amino acids, 78, 176, 202
analgesic essential oils: chamomile German, 73, 79; chamomile Roman, 73, 79; eucalyptus, 73; Italian everlasting, 72; lavender, 73, 79; rose otto, 73, 79; yarrow, 73, 79

anal itch, biochemic cell salts for, 140, 145
anemia, 194–96
antibacterial essential oils: cinnamon, 78; geranium, 73; oregano, 77; rose otto, 73; thyme, 77
anticoagulant essential oils: geranium, 73; Italian everlasting, 72
anti-inflammatory drugs: for adenomyosis, 19; coelomic metaplasia and, 42; growth of endometriosis and, 28; iatrogenic origins of endometriosis and, 42
anti-inflammatory essential oils, 79; chamomile German, 98; chamomile Roman, 98; essential oil blend for, 98; geranium, 73; helichrysum, 72; lavender, 79, 98; peppermint, 98
antioxidants: bioflavonoids, 188; garlic, 61; milk thistle, 110; selenium, 198; turmeric, 55; vitamin C, 186–87; vitamin E, 189. *See also* vitamin C; vitamin E
antiseptic essential oils: geranium, 73; rose otto, 73
antispasmodic essential oils: chamomile Roman, 73; clary sage, 73; geranium, 73, 78; marjoram, 73; rose otto, 73
anxiety, 9; chaste berry for, 107; homeopathic remedies for, 138; vitamin B_5 for, 181

cardamom (*Elettaria cardamomum*): Digestion-Aid Massage Blend, 100–101; Low-Abdominal-Pain Synergy Blend for Hip Massage, 96; tea, for flatulence, 100

CAT or CT scan (computed axial tomography), 16

causes of endometriosis, 21–36; antiestrogen drug Clomid, 27; bath products, 35; coelomic metaplasia, 28–29, 42; congenital or embryonic rest theory, 29–31, 32, 42; corticosteroids, 28; douches, 34–35; environmental pollutants, 43; environmental theories, 31–33; genetic factors, 31; hormonal factors, 29–31, 43; iatrogenic origins, 27–29, 42; immune-system factors, 24–25, 41–42; immunosuppression drugs, 27–28; inflammation, 25–26, 42; interactions of various, 41–43; intestinal parasites, 59; intrauterine migration, 24; lymphatic or vascular transplantation theory (metastasis), 26–29, 42, 68; miscellaneous theories, 33–36; nutrition, poor, 36; prescription drugs, 27–28; retrograde menstruation, 22–24, 41; scientific investigation of, 33; sex during menstruation, 34; STDs, 35, 58–59; stress and emotional factors, 35; tampon use, 34; xenoestrogen overload, 31–32, 43

CDI (color Doppler imaging), 15, 19

cells, 36–39; apoptosis (cell death), 37; calcium and, 200; division called phytohemagglutinin-induced blastogenesis, 186–87; electrochemical factor, 80–81; emotional stress and, 39; estrogen receptors on, 38, 75; metabolism and, 173; neurotransmitters and, 80; nutritional supplements to repair, 39; oxygen and, 38; phytoestrogens and, 38; waste removal from, 38–39; xenoestrogens and, 38

cervix, endometrial cells implanted on, 3

chamomile German (*Matricaria recutita*): as an analgesic, 73, 79; as anti-inflammatory, 98

chamomile Roman (*Anthemis nobilis*), 163; as an analgesic, 73, 79; as anti-inflammatory, 98; as an antispasmodic, 73; calming, in hot water, oil burner, room fragrancer, or diffuser, 105; in Endo Hip Massage Oil Blend, 88; in Endo Hip Massage Oil Blend (Synergistic Blend), 88; in Headache- and Migraine-Cooling Gel, 102–3; as herbal tea, before bedtime, 105

chaste berry (*Vitex agnus castus*), 107–9, 129

Chinese herbs, 126, 129–30; Artemesia vulgaris (mugwort), 134; Dan'e Mixture, 129; keishi-bukuryo-gan, 129; Neiyixiao Recipe, 129. *See also* Chinese medicine

Chinese medicine: acupuncture and acupressure and, 133–35; diagnosis in, 130, 134–35. *See also* Chinese herbs

chlamydia, 17, 58

chlorine: health warnings, 67; in tap water, 64

chocolate, elimination of, 61, 119

chocolate cysts, 4

cholesterol, 54; exercise and regulating, 67; as source of hormones, 53

choline, 185; dietary sources of, 204–8

cinnamon (*Cinnamonum zeylanicum*): as antibacterial, 61, 78; as antiviral, 61, 128

clary sage (*Salvia sclarea*), 164; as antispasmodic, 73; calming, in oil burner, room fragrancer, or diffuser, 105; in Endo Hip Massage Oil Blend, 88; in Endo Hip Massage Oil Blend (Synergistic Blend), 88; in Essential Endo Sitz Bath Blend, 85; in Hot Bath Preparation, 93

cloves, 155; antibacterial properties, 61

coelomic metaplasia, 28–29, 31, 41, 42, 43

coffee, 179; elimination of, 61, 110

cold compresses: for low back pain, 98; for lower abdominal pain, 97; to reduce inflammation, 136

colon: cancer of, 16; sigmoid flexure, endometrial cells implanted on, 3

colonic irrigation, 59
complementary therapies: acupuncture and acupressure, 126, 133–35; "alternative" term, 125; Ayurveda, 126, 130–31; biochemic cell salts, 126, 139–46; bodywork techniques, 126, 131–33; Chinese herbs, 126; choosing a practitioner, 126–27; as diagnostic tools, 126; flower remedies, 126, 146–48; herbalism, 126, 128–30; as holistic, 125–26, 148–50; homeopathy, 126, 137–39; hydrotherapy, 126, 135–36; important considerations, 126–27; as integrative medicine, 126; naturopathy, 126, 148–50; self-help systems, 126; types recommended for endometriosis, 126. *See also specific therapy*
Complete Book of Essential Oils and Aromatherapy, The (Worwood), xiv
congenital or embryonic rest theory, 42
conjugation, 54
constipation, 7, 98–99; biochemic cell salts for, 145, 146; diet and nutrition for, 99; importance of recording, 14; laxatives, cautions against, 99; massage for, 99; painful defecation and, 98; water intake and, 98, 110
coriander (*Coriandrum sativum*), in Digestion-Aid Massage Blend, 100–101
corn, caution for GM products, 60
cortisol, 35
cosmetics, 116–17
cramps. *See* menstrual cramps; pain
CRP (C-reactive protein): inflammation and, 13, 26; testing for, 13
cul-de-sac (adjacent to coccyx): endometrial cells implanted on, 3
culdocentesis, 15
cypress (*Cupressus sempervirens*), 165; in Bloating Synergy Blend for Massage, 94; as a diuretic, 79; in Essential Endo Sitz Bath Blend, 85; for hemorrhoid prevention and relief, 104; in Hot Bath Preparation, 93; for lymph flow, 73
cystoscopy, 15–16
cysts (endometriomas), 4; rupturing, 8; severe stage of endometriosis and, 5

D

dairy products: elimination of, 60, 110; as predominant food, 63
depression, 7, 9; flower remedies for, 147; geranium for, 73; vitamin B5 for, 181
detoxification, 53–55; Ayurveda program for, 131; biochemic cell salts for, 140; body brushing for, 68–72; "body burden" of chemicals, 114; diet and nutrition for, 110; essential oils for, 76; liver health and, 53–55; massage for, 133; milk thistle for, 107, 110; personal care products and, 113–18; substances to avoid, 110; water intake, 55, 110
diabetes: as EFA contraindication, 191; fatigue and, 101; as niacin contraindication, 181
diagnosis of endometriosis: CAT or CT scan, 16; CRP testing, 13; culdocentesis, 15; cystoscopy, 15–16; difficulty of making, 5, 13–18, 47; EBT, 16; examination during menstruation and, 13–14; hormone levels, testing, 29, 47; hysterosalpingography, 16; hysteroscopy, 16; laparoscopy, 13, 15; MRI, 16; need for accurate information about symptoms, 14; other conditions with similar symptoms, 16–17; pattern of symptoms, 13; procedures for, disadvantages of, 15–16; ultrasound, 15
diarrhea, 7, 99–100; biochemic cell salts for, 145; importance of recording, 14
diary or journal: food diary, 62, 209–13; symptom record, 14, 21
diet and nutrition: additives, avoiding, 61–62; balanced, 63; beverages to avoid or eliminate, 61; for constipation relief and prevention, 99; dairy products, elimination of, 60, 110; determining predominant foods in your current diet, 62–63; for detoxification, 110; dietary sources of vitamins and minerals (chart), 204–8; for digestive disorders, 100; elimination of too much fat and sugar, 119;

probiotics, 55, 95, 193–94; purchasing guidelines, 174; repair of cell damage and, 39; selenium, 111, 197–99; testing to determine need for, 174; vitamin A, 176, 177; vitamin B (complex), 111, 176, 177–79; vitamin B_1, 178; vitamin B_2, 180; vitamin B_5, 181–82; vitamin B_6, 108, 111, 182–83; vitamin B_{12}, 183–84; vitamin C, 110, 111, 176, 186–88; vitamin D, 176; vitamin E, 111, 176, 188; vitamin K, 176, 190; water-soluble vitamins, 175, 176; zinc, 111, 196–97

O

oats, 60, 98
obesity, estrogen stored in body fat, 66
onions, 54, 60
orange (*Citrus sinensis*), in Tension-Relieving Blend, 106
orange, as antibacterial, 61
orange blossom herbal tea, 105
oregano (*Origanum vulgare*), 61, 77, 128
ovarian cancer, 16
ovaries, 4; biochemic cell salts for ovarian pain, 144; endometrial cells implanted in, 3, 23; ovarian cysts, 16; ultrasound analysis, 15
ovulation: hormonal imbalance and, 8; new research on, 75; pain and, 8; vitamin B_5 for, 181

P

pain: abdominal, as knifelike, burning, or sharp, 8, 96; abdominal and pelvic, 6, 8, 96; abdominal and pelvic, cold compresses, 97; abdominal and pelvic, importance of recording incidents of, 14; abdominal and pelvic, sitz baths for, 97; adhesions and, 5, 8; backache, 6; backache, heat packs and essential oils, 97–98; cause of endometrial, 72–73; chest area, 6; chronic pelvic, 6; in coccyx, 6; cramps, abdominal, 6, 30, 73; defecation and, 7; degree of, misunder-

stood, 17; degree of, not related to severity of disease, 5, 17–18, 79; dull abdominal or backache, 6; front of thigh, 6; gas pains, 7; headache, 6; histamines and, 8; homeopathic remedies for, 138–39; inflammation and, 53, 72–73; during intercourse (dyspareunia), 5, 6, 9, 48; intermittant pelvic, 6; joint, 6; Low-Abdominal-Pain Synergy Blend for Hip Massage, 96; menstrual, 8; ovulation and, 8; pouch of Douglas and, 43; prostaglandins and, 8; rectal, 6; reducing, research trial on, xiv; rib cage, 6; severity and duration of, 47; shoulder, 6, 15; urinary, 7; vaginal, tampons and, 6. *See also* pain, biochemic cell salts for
pain, biochemic cell salts for: abdominal, as knifelike, burning, or sharp, 144; abdominal and pelvic, 142, 143; backache, 139, 140, 141; bone and joint, 141; cramps, abdominal, 139, 143, 144; cramps, intestinal, 144, 145; ovarian, 144; rectal, 144
parabens, 32–33, 113–14; in antiperspirants/deodorants, 117–18; in cosmetics, 117; names on labels, 114
passiflora, 105
patchouli, 155
peppermint (*Mentha piperita*), 100, 109, 129; as anti-inflammatory, 98; for headaches and migraines, 102–3; in Low-Abdominal-Pain Synergy Blend for Hip Massage, 96; teas, 100, 103, 109
perineal area, 3–4
peritoneum (abdominal cavity), endometrial cells implanted in, 3
personal care products, 113–18; antiperspirants and deodorants, 117–18; chlorine in, 116; cosmetics, 116–17; dioxins in, 116; evaluating for toxins, 113–18; hair products, 116; menstrual care products, 115–16; nail products, 117; parabens in, 32–33, 113–14, 117; phthalates in, 115; sunscreens, 118; tampons, 34, 116

phytoestrogens/phytohormones, 36, 38;
antiquity of use, 75–76; essential oils
as, 74; as natural SERMs, 74–75
PID (pelvic inflammatory disease), 16,
35, 58
Pierson, Roger, 75
pineapple: as anti-inflammatory, 60; as
liver cleanser, 54
pituitary gland, 31; chaste berry and, 108
PMS (premenstrual syndrome), 7, 10;
biochemic cell salts for, 144; chaste
berry for, 107–8; homeopathic remedies for, 138
potassium, 202–3; dietary sources of,
204–8
pouch of Douglas, 4; endometriosis in, 43
probiotics, 55, 94, 193
progesterone: for adenomyosis, 19; balancing, chaste berry for, 108; infertility and, 30; retrograde menstruation
and, 41; synthetic, for endometriosis,
21
prolactin, 108
prostaglandins: and B vitamins, 178;
EFAs and, 190; pain or inflammation
and, 8; type identified in enometrio-
sis (F2-alpha), 30; and vitamin C, 187

R

rectum, 4; biochemic cell salts for pain
in, 144; biochemic cell salts for problems with, 140; bleeding or blood in
stools, 7; endometrial cells implanted
on, 4; pain in, 6
regenerative essential oil, Italian everlasting, 72
retrograde menstruation, 22–24, 41, 42
rice, 60; brown, for detoxification, 55
rose hydrolat, 85
rosemary (*Rosmarinus officinalis*): in
Bloating Synergy Blend for Massage,
94; in Headache- and Migraine-
Cooling Gel, 102–3; as muscle relaxant, 98
rose otto (*Rosa damascena*), 171; as analgesic, 73, 79; as antibacterial, 73; as

antiseptic, 73; complexity and diffi-
culty of producing, 155; in Endo Hip
Massage Oil Blend, 88; in Endo Hip
Massage Oil Blend (Synergistic
Blend), 88; in Essential Endo Sitz
Bath Blend, 85; in Hot Bath Prepara-
tion, 93; for tension relief, 106
rose water, 85

S

sage, as antibacterial, 61
salt, 95; eliminating in diet, 55, 61
Sampson, John A., 22
Schenken, Robert, 24
Schuessler, Wilhelm, 139
Second International Symposium on
Endometriosis, 17
selenium, 111, 197–99
Sexual Chemistry (Grant), 27
sexuality: during Endometriosis Natural
Treatment Program, 113; homeopathic remedies for painful intercourse, 138; importance of recording
activity, 14; pain during intercourse
(dyspareunia), 5, 6, 9, 48, 113; sex during menstruation and endometriosis,
34
sitz baths, 82, 83–87, 136; alternative
method, bath and shower routine,
92–93; alternative method, easy option, 86–87; cold, 84–85; contraindications of, 83; equipment needed for,
84; Essential Endo Sitz Bath Blend,
85; health benefits of, 83, 84; hot, 85;
key elements of, 83–84; special
weekly, 86
skin sensitivity test, 82
smoking: cell damage and, 39; elimination of, 119; nicotine as toxin, 55
Society of Homeopaths, 137
STDs (sexually transmitted diseases):
chlamydia, 17, 58; as cause of endometriosis, 35; genital mycoplasmas,
58–59, 77–78; gonorrhea, 17
stress: bergamot for calming, balancing,
73–74; cellular damage and, 39; as

Valerie Ann Worwood has a doctorate in complementary health and is a clinical aromatherapist who specializes in the natural treatment of female reproductive problems, including endometriosis and infertility. Her books include *The Fragrant Pharmacy*, *The Fragrant Mind*, *The Fragrant Heavens*, and *Aromatherapy for Your Child* (all published in the United Kingdom); and *The Complete Book of Essential Oils and Aromatherapy*, *Aromatherapy for the Healthy Child*, *The Fragrant Mind*, *Essential Aromatherapy*, and *Aromatherapy for the Soul* (all published in the United States).

Julia Stonehouse is a lecturer and writer specializing in reproductive issues and is currently researching the effects of reproduction theory throughout the developing nations. She is author of *Idols to Incubators: Reproduction Theory through the Ages* and a contributor to *Conceiving Persons: Ethnographies of Procreation, Fertility, and Growth*.